OXFORD MEDICAL PUBLICATIONS

....

Evaluating Palliative Care
Establishing the Evidence Base

Evaluating Palliative Care

Establishing the Evidence Base

MARGARET ROBBINS

Research Fellow, Department of Palliative Medicine
University of Bristol

OXFORD   NEW   YORK   TOKYO
OXFORD UNIVERSITY PRESS
1998

Oxford University Press, Great Clarendon Street, Oxford OX2 6DP

Oxford New York
Athens Auckland Bangkok Bogota Bombay
Buenos Aires Calcutta Cape Town Dar es Salaam
Delhi Florence Hong Kong Istanbul Karachi
Kuala Lumpur Madras Madrid Melbourne
Mexico City Nairobi Paris Singapore
Taipei Tokyo Toronto Warsaw

and associated companies in
Berlin Ibadan

Oxford is a trade mark of Oxford University Press

Published in the United States
by Oxford University Press Inc., New York

A catalogue record for this book is available from the British Library

Library of Congress Cataloging in Publication Data
Robbins, Margaret, Dr.
Evaluating palliative care : establishing the evidence base /
Margaret Robbins
(Oxford medical publications)
Includes bibliographical references and index.
1. Palliative treatment. 2. Hospice care. I. Title.
II. Series.
[DNLM: 1. Palliative Care. 2. Terminal Care. 3. Quality
Assurance Health Care. WB 310 R 635e 1998]
R726.8.R63 1998   362.1'75–dc21   97-42665
ISBN 0 19 262621 3 (Pbk)

Typeset by Downdell, Oxford
Printed in Great Britain by
Biddles Ltd
Guildford & King's Lynn

Preface

The idea for this book arose from a frustration at not finding a text that brought together the methodological issues which I perceived faced health services researchers in the field of palliative care, particularly in relation to carrying out evaluation research. Since the inception of the book, I have come across a number of excellent reviews of different aspects of palliative care research, but still nothing that brings the strands together—that is what I aim to do in this book. By considering evaluation in both its widest and narrowest sense, and by trying to understand how the effectiveness of a disparate service like palliative care could be assessed, I have brought together a number of themes which commonly face the novice palliative care researcher. My viewpoint and choice of literature has been influenced by several concerns, including the dilemmas of health care purchasing, public health medicine, and increasingly, the challenge that whatever it is, it has to be 'evidence based'.

I hope that this book will be of use to health service researchers and clinicians interested in carrying out applied research. It was never conceived to be a clinical textbook; that niche is very well filled by the *Oxford textbook of palliative medicine* and others which aim to educate the practitioner in the different skills and concerns of palliative care. I am not a palliative care provider, being neither clinician, social worker, counsellor, nor cleric. My training is instead in social anthropology and I have spent the last decade researching various aspects of care for the dying and the bereaved. Of the projects I have been involved in, at least a few have been evaluations of palliative care. I probably consider myself to be what Professor David Clark has recently described himself to be—a 'critical friend'.[1] That is, not an insider, but not an entirely impartial outsider either.

This is not a 'systematic review' of the research literature. That term has developed a precise meaning (and method) recently, and I cannot pretend to have scoured all the relevant journals published

---

[1] 'A critical friend? Some personal reflections on research in palliative care.' Paper presented by David Clark to the South and West Palliative Care Research Network meeting, 30 June 1997, Southampton, UK.

over the last 25 years. Neither have I systematically classified each research report in terms of the quality of the effectiveness evidence. I have however covered a great deal of the palliative care literature, not confining my reading to reports of studies of certain types. Much relevant material has been found in reviews, personal views, clinical case histories, and the more philosophical texts on death and dying. It is worth pointing out that I have not investigated the vast literature on the palliative and terminal care needs of children with life-limiting illness.

Evaluation, as a distinct activity within the field of health service research, has not received as much critical attention as it deserves. An evaluation study is more than tacking some hastily thought-out recommendations to the end of a conventional research report. Many people believe that to make evaluation research properly useful to those it concerns, the barriers between the researcher and the researched have to be broken down. Without practitioner ownership of the research, and involvement in the negotiation of its parameters and outcome indicators, there is little reason to wonder why findings do not get taken up in practice. The main message that I would like to convey through this book is that palliative care evaluation has to be a creative activity, requiring multidisciplinary skills, in full awareness of the political context in which it is being conducted. The social and clinical sciences have a tremendous variety of perspectives and methods of relevance to the evaluation of health services; it would be regrettable if concentration on the three 'E's of effectiveness, efficiency, and economy, was at the expense of ignoring the three 'A's of appropriateness, acceptability, and accessibility.

Bristol   M.R.
December 1997

Acknowledgements

This book is based on the experiences of reading, writing, and teaching over several years spent in three different university departments. In the process I have drawn from the knowledge and insights of many people, and each department has influenced my thinking and given it a particular flavour. It was whilst working in the Department of Social Medicine at the University of Bristol that the idea for the book was conceived. The first draft was completed and commented on by Pat Jackson and Stephen Frankel. My focus on health services research broadened while I worked in the School of Social Sciences at the University of Bath. I would like to thank the undergraduates of the B.Sc. in Social Policy and Administration who attended my lectures on social policy evaluation—I think I learned as much from them as they did from me. Finally, my present colleagues in the Department of Palliative Medicine at the University of Bristol have provided a much-needed anchor to the real world of palliative care research. I am particularly grateful to Geoffrey Hanks who has read and commented on drafts of the chapters, and to the various palliative care service providers, patients and families whom I have encountered during my research endeavours. Thanks are also due to the funders of these projects, including the Medical Research Council, the Wellcome Trust, the NHS South and West Research and Development Directorate, the Nuffield Foundation, and St Peter's Hospice, Bristol.

I am indebted to my husband, Ben Toth, who has constantly provided encouragement, criticism, and inspiration throughout the time of writing and rewriting. Our young daughters, Hyat and Mary, have just survived the process and I thank them for their forbearance.

The staff at Oxford University Press are to be commended for their success in extracting the manuscript from me.

To Peter and Betty

Contents

1

Evaluation: what is it and why do it?

Introduction

'There is often a serenity—sometimes even a dignity—in the act of death, but rarely in the process of dying' (Nuland 1997). This quotation from Sherwin Nuland's book, *How we die*, suggests by implication the scale of the task facing those members of the caring professions who support dying people on their way to death. In past centuries, the *ars moriendi*, or the art of dying, was both a religious and cultural endeavour; a 'good' death uplifted the souls of family and friends who gathered round the deathbed of a person who had probably succumbed to a rapidly life-threatening illness. Nowadays, the art of dying has perhaps been replaced by the art of saving lives. Although much of modern medicine aims to prevent or cure serious illness, its effect can as well be to postpone death in such a way that the dying stage becomes lengthened. A 'good' death is considered by many to be a quick departure from the world, preferably during sleep, or possibly after a very short illness (Payne *et al.* 1996). For increasing numbers of the population however, death does not come suddenly. Figures suggest that up to 50 per cent of all deaths are anticipated in some way (National Council for Hospice and Specialist Palliative Care Services (NCHSPCS) 1995*a*).

While many would like to believe that an anticipated death can nevertheless be a dignified death (given the capacity of modern health care to be so effective at preventing it), Nuland suggests that time and time again modern health care in fact offers quite the opposite (Nuland 1997). This observation has been made frequently, and it was primarily due to the recognition that people with cancer were particularly likely to be 'abandoned' by curative medicine to a time of painful deterioration and death, that the hospice and palliative care movement developed so rapidly from the 1960s.

The expansion, proliferation, and differentiation of palliative care provision in the UK, North America, Australasia, and indeed worldwide, has been well described and discussed (see, for example, Saunders 1993). In many ways, the process of expansion of the palliative care sector has been similar to general trends within the fields of clinical practice and health care policy. Many areas of patient care, like palliative care, have seen an increased emphasis on multidisciplinary team work, the harnessing of psychosocial and complementary therapies, and holistic assessment. And many areas of social welfare, as well as health provision, have placed more stress on what is termed the 'mixed economy' of care (Spicker 1995). With their substantial reliance on charitable funding and extensive use of volunteers, many palliative care services illustrate the complexities of integrating statutory sector provision with voluntary and informal sector provision. In addition, palliative care services face the same demands for evidence of effectiveness and value for money as do general health services.

Many forms of clinical care have persisted over the years without proper assessment of their effectiveness while underassessed interventions and technologies have been introduced with considerable implications for health care spending. In the early 1990s it was widely reported that only around 20 per cent of health service interventions had ever been formally evaluated (Consumer Health Information Consortium 1994). The figure may underestimate the number of interventions that have been subject to clinical trial; but there is a strong feeling that more can be known about the effectiveness of services, and that more can be done to disseminate findings. In recent years strong pressure has come from the central National Health Service (NHS) Executive in the UK, and government agencies in other countries for the planning and purchasing of health care to be based explicitly on clear evidence of need and effectiveness (Department of Health 1993). In the UK, these ideas have been put into action by the establishment of a National Research and Development Directorate, whose brief is to commission high-quality research, support training in health care research, and ensure the maximum impact of research findings on the organization and delivery of health care (Department of Health 1993). In addition, the establishment of the International Cochrane Collaboration is a significant contribution to the development of evidence-based practice. This collaboration supports the systematic review of evidence for a wide range of clinical interventions, and encourages the dissemination of the results.

All forms of quality assurance, audit, social and financial accounting have become more important over the past 35 to 40 years with the increasing scale and complexity of organizations and public sector services. The emergence of a distinct field of applied research—evaluation research—to address questions of effectiveness and efficiency can be traced back to the 1960s and 70s. Much of the early development of evaluation theory took place in North America where a concern to assess the impact of various state-funded educational and social programmes spawned an evaluation profession, with specialist research status and associated literature, and an academic career ladder (Weiss and Rein 1969; Cronbach 1982).

Within the health sciences, under the influence of the emerging schools of management and operational research, more formal evaluation of health care effectiveness was seen as important to run alongside the well-established tradition of biomedical basic research (Holland 1983). During the 1980s escalating health care costs brought a need across North America and Europe for ways to contain such expenditure. Policy makers were increasingly faced with rationing decisions, relating both to the volume and type of health care provision. Pressures to demonstrate the effectiveness not only of health care innovations but also of existing procedures and services derived principally from the perceived need to use limited health care funds in the most efficient and effective way possible; particularly so given the ageing profile of Western populations, the relentless development of expensive, high-technology medical therapies, and a better-informed public with higher expectations.

Evaluation is clearly a form of applied research which is designed to answer current concerns or questions about the functioning or impact of services, programmes, or policies. It is about using the tools and techniques developed in primary or basic research, and applying them to questions of need, effectiveness, efficiency, appropriateness, and acceptability. Whereas basic research is supposed to be (although not always believed to be) value free, evaluation research is quite the opposite; in fact it probably works best when it explicitly embraces the particular values or norms of a specific orientation or political stance. Essentially, evaluation is concerned with establishing the 'value' or 'worth' of a service, programme, or policy. And to determine value, there have to concepts and norms against which the value is assessed. In practice then, evaluation research goes beyond the mere reporting of facts and figures to a judgement on their meaning for the service or policy under consideration. In this sense, evaluation has emerged as a tool to be used by health service planners, managers, and policymakers to support decision making.

The extent to which palliative care policy and practice has been evaluated is the subject of this book. Three main purposes lie behind this endeavour. The first is to lay out the results of evaluations of palliative care and to draw attention to the rather meagre evidence base. The second is to provide a resource for anybody undertaking an evaluation of palliative care services, or who is involved in using the results of evaluations in the planning or development of palliative care. The third purpose is to contribute to the theory and methodology of evaluation research. A tremendous amount of evaluation research is carried out, at substantial cost to the health services, and by using palliative care as an example, the strength, the weaknesses, and also the limitations of evaluative enterprise will be explored. An interplay between what the research literature reveals about the nature of palliative care, and what palliative care reveals about the task and mission of evaluation forms a constant theme throughout the book. Research studies from various countries (particularly the United States, Canada, Australia, New Zealand, and Europe) are drawn upon, but the greatest proportion of research evidence considered emanates from the UK. It is anticipated however, that the general points will be applicable to researchers working in a range of contexts and settings, as well as in other areas of broadly based care.

This chapter is concerned essentially with the mechanics of evaluation research. Although there are a number of specialist texts on evaluation research to which the reader is referred (for example, Rossi and Freeman 1993; St Leger *et al.* 1992), the chapter begins with an overview of the steps that are commonly taken to perform an evaluation, and examines the reasons why evaluations are carried out and what research methods are appropriate for the different purposes. The case of palliative care research is then presented, focusing on some of the difficulties which are frequently encountered in defining and conceptualizing this area of care. This overview provides a theoretical and methodological structure for the following four chapters which discuss in detail the scope and focus of research with the recipients and providers of palliative care. The final chapter attempts to anchor the discussion in the real world of research and policymaking, and proposes a framework for future evaluation research in palliative care.

Approaches to evaluation

The field of evaluation research is of course extremely wide and varied since evaluations are carried out for many purposes. An organization or service may undertake an evaluation due to external pressure (from government, from regulatory bodies, or from commissioning agencies) or internal pressure (to assess current working practices or the impact of change, for example). An organization may wish to assess the impact of a service after a certain length of time, in order to review the advisability of its continuation, or it may be more interested in the incremental development of a service, using an ongoing system of monitoring and feedback to foster good practice. Some evaluations may hinge on the comparison of services in different geographical areas; others may focus on comparisons over time within the one service under consideration. In the field of hospice and palliative care there are examples of all of these kinds of evaluation. Large-scale evaluations, for example the National Hospice Study of 1978–85 in the USA (Mor *et al.* 1988), have sought to compare hospice care with conventional care. Small-scale evaluations have aimed to chart the satisfaction of patients and their families with the services of a specific hospice home care service over time (Doyle 1991).

There have been several attempts to categorize different kinds of evaluations with their different purposes. The first handbook in the Program Evaluation Kit published by Sage in the late 1980s sets out a framework of different approaches to evaluation (Stecher and Davis 1987):

1. The experimental approach to evaluation seeks to apply the principles of experimental science, with the aim of producing generalizable conclusions about the outcome of a particular service through the control of variables and simplification of the question under scrutiny. This kind of evaluation has more in common with basic biomedical research, with its emphasis on analytic methods

resulting in quantitative data. Employing this approach, an experimental design using random allocation to the intervention and control groups is considered to be superior, but where randomization is not possible, then the internal validity of quasi-experimental approaches can be enhanced through statistical modelling.

2. The goal-oriented approach sets out to investigate the success of a service in meeting specific goals and objectives that have been set for the service. These goals may not be applicable to other services elsewhere and so the evaluation may not seek to produce generalizable findings. In many ways, this approach to evaluation shares some of the features of clinical audit, and follows its cyclical path.

3. Another approach to evaluation is that which focuses upon the most relevant information that can be used for making decisions about the management and operation of services. This decision making approach requires close liaison with the staff involved in the planning and delivery of services, not just at the outset but as the services become established. Again this kind of approach is tailored to the circumstances surrounding the specific service being evaluated, and only the most general aspects of the evaluation may have wider applicability.

4. The user-oriented approach focuses upon the participation of service providers in the evaluation to increase the likelihood of the evaluation's findings being acted upon and used. Involving staff in the planning and execution of evaluations mean that they become part of the inquiry process—not simply passive subjects of an investigation. The idea of user involvement (also called 'stakeholder evaluation') has a longer history in the field of social programme evaluation than health care evaluation (Ferman 1969; Smith and Cantley 1985), although 'ownership' of research has been seen as important for the successful implementation of clinical guidelines. Because the user is involved in this approach, evaluations can be subjected to a variety of pressures, particularly relating to redirection of the research according to user preferences and interests.

5. The responsive approach to evaluation attempts to understand an issue from as many points of view as possible. Using naturalistic methods, the aim is to portray the multidimensional and complex webs of interaction and relationship that characterize the organization and delivery of the service in question. This method is typified

by qualitative data collection, mainly from observation and inter-viewing. Although it is probably impossible to take into account all the perspectives of all interested parties, the strengths of this approach lie in its capacity to identify problems, particularly ones which had not been anticipated, while its weakness lies in the difficulty of simplifying information for the purposes of decision making.

Many other types of evaluation have been identified (see Robson 1993), but perhaps the most widely used distinction is that between the formative and summative approaches. Formative evaluation is intended to improve the development of a service or programme, while summative evaluation focuses upon effectiveness and the meeting of goals. The distinction between the two approaches is not clear cut, since a formative evaluation can have summative elements, and a summative evaluation can have formative effects on future developments of the service. A similar distinction is also often made between outcome and process evaluation. An emphasis on the impact or outcome of a service solely in terms of the extent to which it has achieved its goals or objectives, is likely to provide an impoverished account of the overall impact of a service in relation to both its intended and unintended consequences. Process evaluation is concerned therefore with how services are delivered ('what actually happens') and so would constitute an important aspect of both the summative and formative approaches.

Both formative and summative approaches to evaluation have been used in the field of palliative care. Addington-Hall's study of the effect of palliative care co-ordinators on patient quality of life can be regarded as a summative evaluation since the focus was on measuring the effect of the new service after a fixed length of time in relation to the stated objectives (Addington-Hall *et al.* 1992). In contrast, Dand's evaluation of client satisfaction with care at the Leicestershire Hospice can be considered to be a formative evalu-ation, since the main purpose was to examine satisfaction with the process of care from the perspectives of the patients and family carers, and to provide feedback for improving communication and patient care within the service (Dand *et al.* 1991).

There can be a number of other considerations which shape the choice of evaluation approach and contribute to the nature of an evaluation project. Whether the evaluation is commissioned or not (and by whom) is important. An evaluation which is part of a national programme of commissioned research may have to conform to a specific methodology and orientation, while an evaluation commissioned by a local agency (for example, a hospice) might be negotiated in more detail between the researchers and the funder. When an evaluation is not commissioned as such, but arises from the interests of a research group (often university based), then more freedom is exercised over the type of evaluation approach adopted and the status of the subsequent results. Who actually carries out the evaluation is also an important factor. Evaluations which are carried out by external researchers (that is, non-service providers or employees) without sustained engagement with the service stake-holders (practitioners, managers, clients/patients, and so on) may be less successful at capturing the process aspects. There is a clear difference between research carried out by external agencies where the priority is to collect objective data for measuring the effectiveness of the service provision, and research carried out in a collaborative manner, with sensitivity to the perspectives of the various stakeholders, even encouraging their participation in the research process and fostering a spirit of self-evaluation. The time-scale over which the evaluation is carried out is also a major consideration. When results are needed urgently then certain types of research will not be possible. It is probably true that in evaluation research, more so than basic clinical or biomedical research, there is enhanced pressure to produce results quickly, with the concomitant dangers of incomplete or insufficient data gathering and analysis.

Practical steps to evaluation

Evaluations can be carried out to address questions of technical effectiveness; they may be designed to illuminate innovatory practice by service providers; or they may aim to open up a subject to debate and to the introduction of change. Whatever the purpose however, each evaluation should try to describe clearly what a service is, or what an organization is trying to achieve; to assess how far it is succeeding (and at what cost); to identify problematic areas (or unexpected consequences) of service delivery or organization performance; and crucially to draw broader lessons for policy-makers, planners, managers, and practitioners. Many would characterize evaluation research as the *systematic collection* of evidence in a rigorous manner, combined with the entering into *dialogue* with the various parties or stakeholders involved, in order to identify with, and speak to their different political interests and preoccupations (Room 1986).

The steps to carrying out an evaluation are essentially the same as those for any research project. The skills involved are the same. Where an evaluation project differs from a basic or 'pure' science project is that attention is directed to practical problems or questions involving services and programmes, rather than simply gaining knowledge (discovering truths) or developing and testing theory. Evaluation research is also more likely to use a combination of research methods, rather than plough a single methodological (and epistemological) furrow. The steps which will be discussed in turn are the clarification and application of aims and objectives; the choice of appropriate research design; and the dissemination of results.

Setting aims and objectives

Clarifying the aims and objectives of an evaluation study is a vital first step. In general an aim can be thought of as an overriding purpose for the evaluation, for example, 'to assess the effectiveness of hospice care'. The objectives go a step further and propose how the overall aim of the assessment can be put into operation: for example, 'to assess the effectiveness of hospice care in relation to patient quality of life, family carer satisfaction, and cost of inpatient care'. This process begins to establish, both explicitly and implicitly, the criteria by which achievement of the aim will be judged. For example, a preoccupation with outcome (and effectiveness) may well become apparent at this stage.

Since evaluation has become an important activity for the demonstration of accountability in the use of public, private, or charitable funds, then it is clear that the potential exists for evaluations to become politically and ideologically charged— particularly in a context of competition between services for limited funds. Every evaluation is done for a particular reason, with a particular audience in mind. And each evaluation will tend to take on board an agenda which will serve as the yardstick (the set of values) against which the results will be compared (St Leger *et al.* 1992). Currently, there are a number of 'agendas' which appear to provide such criteria for health care evaluation studies. Dowie (1996) identifies these as the movements of evidence-based medicine; cost-effectiveness; and patient and public preferences. The boundaries between the three are blurred, but each has a particular focus. The evidence-based medicine movement (EBM) is concerned with the adoption by clinicians of a willingness to learn and apply objective empirical evidence about the effect of procedures (Sackett and Rosenburg 1995). The cost-effectiveness movement starts with the proposition that costs represent foregone benefits to other patients, and so clinical decision making needs to be carried out in full cognizance of the resource constraints of health services. The patient and public preferences movement emphasizes the need for clinicians to take account of patient and societal preferences in clinical decision making. It is clear that each of these three areas of concern will tend to drive a certain kind of evaluation study. The paradigm of evidence-based medicine (or practice) will tend to encourage evaluations which focus on relatively narrow questions of therapeutic effectiveness and which will need to adopt experimental research designs in order to produce the desired quality of evidence. A concern with cost-effectiveness will tend to encourage evaluations of service efficiency, possibly widening out to cover equity in access to health care, as well as the more classical forms of economic evaluation. Taking into account patient and public preference will lead to a focus on satisfaction with care, participation in decision making, and utility values.

Returning to the example already proposed of an evaluation of the effectiveness of hospice care—the objectives proposed reflect elements from all these major concerns in health care evaluation. For the purposes of the final analysis, it will be necessary however to choose one of the objectives to provide the primary outcome indicator.

Appropriate research designs for evaluation

Much of the evaluation of welfare and educational programmes in the USA and the UK in the 1960s and 70s, initially used an approach which drew heavily on experimental research methods. More recently, other research methodologies have been used in recognition of the fact that experimental and quasi-experimental methods are overly rigid in the assessment of broad-based services, as characterized by multiple outcomes and uncontrolled levels of variables (states which are dependent on social circumstances and institutional arrangements). Evaluation in the health services has been slower to take on board the range of methods that are available to evaluation research. Many aspects of health care which have been subject to summative evaluation concern interventions of a relatively fixed character, such as drug and vaccine tests, new types of surgery, and certain diagnostic developments. Here, the randomized controlled trial methods derived from R. A. Fisher's classic work on agricultural experiments have tended to be adopted. However, many health care interventions are neither so focused in their effect nor contained in the process of their delivery; they are bound up with interprofessional relationships, locally developed health care systems, and varying levels of investment, and have varying effects amongst patients with differing socio-economic, cultural, and educational backgrounds. For these kinds of service or programme, summative or outcome evaluations are not well served by experimental research methods, especially if they are used alone (Pope and Mays 1995).

The aims and objectives of an evaluation will of course have a strong influence on the research strategy that will most appropriate. In general, there are three main research strategies that are widely used in social and health research. The experimental (and quasi-experimental) method measures the effect of manipulating one variable upon another variable. The survey method collects information in a standardized form from groups of people. The case-study method involves the accumulation of detailed, intensive knowledge about a single 'case' or a small number of related cases (Robson 1993). There are as well a number of data-collection methods or tactics which can be utilized within each general research strategy: questionnaires (administered and self-report); observation (direct and indirect or unobtrusive); interviews (formal and informal); collection and analysis of documentary evidence. Finally, data may be collected and analysed according to either the conventions of the deductive scientific method or the inductive methods of naturalistic inquiry. For a detailed discussion of research design, methods, and analysis, the reader is referred to Robson (1993) as a comprehensive introductory text.

Different evaluation approaches do tend to draw on specific research strategies, but crucially the evaluation question itself will determine the appropriate strategy, or combination of strategies, to use. The quantitative / qualitative debate which dominated methodological discourse through the 1980s has now largely been replaced by 'multimethodism' (see for example, Carey 1993; and Holman 1993). Experimental methods of research have been criticized for oversimplification, artificiality, and control (McGourty 1993), emphasizing internal validity at the expense of producing information useful for service improvement, while advocates of qualitative methods, which can better cope with diversity and multiple perspectives, have failed to deal with the issue of validity in a way that is wholly convincing to planners and decision makers (Chen 1988).

Multimethod evaluation research, which draws on the strengths of different methods and thereby counterbalances their respective weaknesses (Ong 1993), has become more commonplace. Health services research, for example, is conceptualized as a multidisciplinary activity with epidemiologists, medical statisticians, health economists, sociologists, anthropologists, and psychologists working together with clinicians to bring their disciplinary epistemologies to bear on questions of health service effectiveness. Although the randomized controlled trial has risen to occupy a prominent place in the range of methods for evaluating therapeutic effect, its application is widely accepted to be limited by numerous ethical and practical difficulties, while its potential use in the assessment of the quality (as opposed to the effectiveness) of care is circumscribed (Orchard 1994). To answer the wider questions asked by health service planners, providers, and policymakers, the randomized controlled trial needs to be complemented by economic, social, and process (health care delivery) evaluation.

The good evaluator is one who is able to select a technique or combination of techniques that are appropriate to the given situation, in full understanding of the aims of the evaluation and any theoretical perspective which has been adopted. Very frequently, an evaluation will use a hybrid of research methods, particularly when it is important to investigate process and outcome factors. However, such an approach, while adding to the completeness and validity of the results, inevitably adds to the time and other resources required, and will be considerably more demanding in terms of complexity of analysis than single-method research. The costs of answering the different levels or hierarchies of questions will need to be weighed up. Researchers who have attempted multimethod research report that data analysis is arduous and intensive (Corner 1991), not only because the process of setting data collected by one method against others is practically complex, but also because the philosophical backgrounds to the different methods of data collection produce incongruities.

Multimethod research can be carried out in different ways, and involves different degrees of sophistication. It can be a relatively *ad hoc* exercise, used to ensure completeness of information gathering, or an exercise underpinned by a set of guiding principles. Its main advantage is in permitting triangulation. In navigation, triangulation is a method of finding out where something is by getting a 'fix' on it in relation to a number of other known points. Using this process in research involves attempting to ensure the validity of a set of findings by using different data sources, methods, theory, or investigator (Denzin 1988; Norman *et al.* 1992). While in many ways triangulation appears to involve the same processes as those described by Ong in relation to multimethod research (Ong 1993), it is more focused on the assessment of the validity of results achieved through different means (Huberman and Miles 1994), rather than simply a bringing together of methodologies which contrast with one another for the sake of variety or which are tacked on to a study for the sake of 'political correctness'.

Dissemination of results

Evaluation research differs from basic research in that the evaluator him or herself is likely to enter the political fray when the results are produced and published. Evaluations are carried out in social and political contexts, with multiple stakeholders. The providers of a service being evaluated may well feel strongly about the content and presentation of the evaluation results, particularly if their own performance is being held up to public scrutiny. If the results of a summative evaluation are likely to lead to cut-backs in funding or the discontinuation of a programme, then the dissemination of results has to handled with extreme caution.

These points suggest that dissemination of findings has to be planned for right at the beginning of an evaluation project. Indeed, to maintain co-operation with those being evaluated, regular feedback during the research period may be important both to maintain interest in the project and to allow a measure of participation. The strength of collaborative evaluation, involving partnership and participation in the research process, instils ownership of evaluation findings with the resultant greater likelihood of their use for reflection and action (Traylen 1994).

A general feature of evaluation research is the production of recommendations for future action. Robson (1993) suggests that it is most important that recommendations should be clearly derived from the data presented in the evaluation report, and that they should also be practical. Relating back to the points already made about collaborative research, the negotiation of recommendations with the decision makers, or whoever is going to use the evaluation findings, is likely to increase the chance that they will be acted upon. Again, this process will be influenced by the status of the evaluator; whether he or she (or the team) are outsiders to the organization or service, or not.

Does evaluation change practice?

The extent to which change is actually initiated by the results of an evaluation is only slightly in the control of the evaluator. As a result of over 40 years of work in the field of programme evaluation in the United States, Cronbach (1982) concluded that the results of evaluations only partially influence resource allocation and decision making. This is an important point to keep in mind in assessing the impact of evaluation research in health services generally and in the field of palliative care in particular. Evaluators need to accept that their efforts are part of a complex mosaic from which actions and decisions emerge. Palliative care provision may be influenced by the results of evaluation, it may be influenced as well by the impact of national health policies and politics, local health district purchasing priorities, and also by the policies of the national cancer charities.

It is often observed that there can be a regrettable lack of impact of the results of even well-conducted research. Many evaluation reports do indeed appear to end up being used as door props or gathering dust at the back of shelves. More attention is however being directed to best practice in the dissemination and implementation of findings, and indeed, to enhancing the cost-effectiveness of research (Buxton and Hanney 1996). A number of models of research utilization in practice have been identified which can be broadly divided into those which are likely to give rise to pessimism, and those which will encourage optimism. The models which will tend to produce pessimism are those which assume that there is a linear relationship between the posing of a problem, its investigation by research, and its solution through the application of the research findings. Because it is observed repeatedly that problems do not disappear, despite the research, it is pessimistically felt that all research is likely to be similarly ignored or doomed. The optimist, on the other hand, is more likely to be satisfied with the 'limestone' model of research utilization (Weiss 1979). New information and knowledge percolates through the political environment in a diffused pattern, over an unpredictable time-scale. Just as water falling upon a limestone cliff will eventually trickle out at the bottom, perhaps through unexpected channels, so research findings may be taken up in surprising ways, and have a diffused rather than direct impact upon subsequent practice. What might hasten and intensify this process is the way in which research results are disseminated and, for example, the extent to which the media becomes interested in them, and how accessible they are to the various networks of policy- and decision makers.

Palliative care and evaluation

The purpose of this book is to examine questions of evaluation as they relate to the care of people who are ill, and reaching the end of their lives. Referring to people as being 'terminally ill' has become a shorthand way of describing a specific set of circumstances; that is, that any active therapy being received is not being offered with curative intent, physical deterioration has come to affect everyday functioning, the deterioration has become progressive and irreversible, and that survival is likely to be counted in weeks and months rather than years. The phrase 'terminally ill' is used therefore to describe the life span stage of the kind of person who may require palliative care, although, of course, the principles and approach of palliative care may well be appropriate to many caring situations which do not involve the kind of terminal illness just described. This book primarily is about palliative care as offered to those with a specific constellation of health, social, and psychological requirements relating to the relative imminence of their death.

In common with other specialties and professional groupings, increasing pressure is being felt within the multidisciplinary field of specialist palliative care for evidence demonstrating the effectiveness, appropriateness, and acceptability of services (Higginson 1992; Clark 1993*a*; McQuay and Moore 1994; NCHSPCS 1995*b*). Palliative care is a broad activity with medical, nursing, and supportive care coming from a variety of specialties and sectors, and attempts to evaluate the effectiveness of the specialist services (that is, those services specifically set up to care for people who are terminally ill, often those with cancer) have faced a number of methodological and practical problems (Goddard 1993; Higginson 1997; Rinck *et al.* 1997). These problems are essentially those that face other health care practitioners—setting standards in care, developing valid and reliable methods of assessing those standards, and being able to use research findings to inform policy and practice.

Defining palliative care

A definition of palliative care, and an understanding of what is provided and how, is pivotal in any type of evaluation. It is important to be able to isolate the field of palliative care, so that it can be evaluated as an area of activity which is distinct from other forms of nursing, medical, and supportive care. This is not an easy task however, although guidance from the NCHSPCS has been offered. It suggests that distinctions can be made between the following terms: palliative care; palliative care services; the palliative care approach; palliative medicine; specialist palliative care services; hospice and hospice care; and terminal care (NCHSPCS 1995*a*). Other definitions concentrate on the difference between the palliative approach, palliative interventions, and specialist palliative care (Finlay and Jones 1995).

Not only have the services offered by specialist providers of palliative care such as hospices spread from the confines of hospice programmes into mainstream care through hospital liaison nurses, palliative care teams, and hospice-at-home schemes, but many nonspecialist health care professionals apply the principles of palliative care during their routine work, and many indeed hold specialist qualifications in palliative care, care of the dying, bereavement care, and counselling. *The Oxford textbook of palliative medicine*, which makes a distinction between palliative medicine as the medical specialty practised by doctors and palliative care as the care offered by a multidisciplinary team of health and social work professionals in addition to volunteers, suggests a number of definitions which can be summarized into the following three main principles (Doyle *et al.* 1993):

1. Palliative care is a philosophy of care both for people who are dying and those who look after them.
2. Palliative care is a set of expert clinical practices in physical symptom management and control.
3. Palliative care is a set of expert counselling practices for the relief of suffering and distress.

It is asserted that what makes palliative care different from standard medical and nursing care is the integration of these three elements: the emphasis on caring for the mind, body, and spirit, and an attitude to life and death which refuses to see death as 'a medical defeat or, worse still, a statistical embarrassment' (Doyle *et al.* 1993).

Palliative care as a philosophy of care

One of the most useful ways of defining palliative care is as a philosophy or an approach. The hallmarks of the palliative care approach are an openness and honesty about dealing with the reality of dying and death; a commitment to assessing the total comfort care needs of patients and their close family or friends; and the will to address these needs through the proactive involvement of other professionals in other settings (instilling in each palliative care professional a commitment to teamwork and effective communication).

As a specialist form of care, this holistic approach is formalized through interdisciplinary teamwork (Ajemian 1993*a*). Ideally a team is composed of physicians to alleviate pain and other physical symptoms, nurses to offer comfort and physical care, social workers to address practical caring problems in the household and give emotional support, chaplains to provide religious services and facilitate spiritual or existential discussions, and other therapists to help enhance the quality of daily life. Volunteers as well can have a role in the interdisciplinary team—possibly meeting a family during a time of terminal illness and carrying on their contact into the time of bereavement.

The philosophy of palliative care and the specialist practise of it can, however, be conceptually and practically separated. Many clinicians use a palliative care approach as previously outlined but are not accredited specialists in palliative care. Indeed, much of the philosophy of palliative care overlaps with general principles of good clinical practice. However, a goal of the palliative care 'movement' is to attain a situation where the philosophy of palliative care informs the approach and practice of all clinicians working with people who are terminally ill. This being the case, the question can be asked as to how a specialist sector can become part and parcel of routine clinical care? Figure 1.1 presents a model of how many specialist palliative care clinicians may be working, both as specialists and as educators, with their non-specialist colleagues.

This model of the relationship between the specialist and non-specialist sector is essentially dynamic, since local situations, resources, and personnel rapidly change. Such changes necessitate a continuing need for a specialist sector to keep disseminating

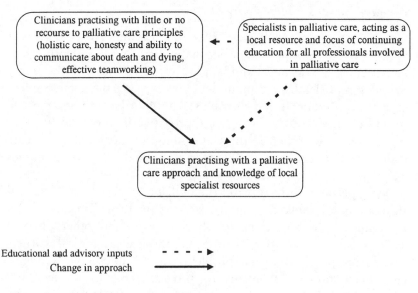

Fig. 1.1   Model of the relationship between specialist and non-specialist sectors of palliative care.

principles of good general palliative care practice, to act as a continually updated specialist resource giving advice and practical support to non-specialists, and to provide the education and training which raise the general standards of palliative care amongst all clinicians. This model is predicated upon a number of assumptions about the way in which non-specialist clinicians work. For example, it is assumed that many clinicians face time and resource constraints that limit the ideal standard of care which they would wish to offer to terminally ill patients with acute problems; and it is also assumed that many clinicians, despite the nature of their work, do have difficulties in coping and communicating with people who are facing dying and death. A specialty interest in palliative care can help to maintain high professional standards, support non-specialists in their more difficult cases, and generally keep a high profile for this kind of approach to patient care.

Defining palliative care as an approach to patient care is a useful first step in teasing out what is meant by the term. Clearly, palliative care is not just about hospices, Macmillan nurses, and the other institutions and forms of care which have become synonymous with the specialist palliative care sector. It is about an attitude to patient care which in many cases may not even involve the utilization of any specialist palliative care interventions.

Is this approach to patient care new? It is sometimes argued that palliative care represents a rediscovery of a set of attitudes to dying and death which were held before the advent of 'modern medicine' with its cure-oriented focus. However, others argue that patterns of disease, with their social and cultural representations, have moved on too far in the intervening 60-odd years for latent attitudes to be reawakened. Walter, for example, argues that contemporary or 'neo-modern' death (Walter's term) is quite dissimilar to traditional death, in that the dying trajectory is generally more prolonged; meaning that many people are, for some considerable time, conscious of the fact that they are dying. In addition, because life is less rooted in community, death has become a private, more individualistic experience, with a greater emphasis on personal choice and being able to die in one's chosen way (Walter 1994). Walter's comparisons of attitudes to death over time suggest that palliative care is very much a product of the late twentieth century, and represents part of a more general movement towards holistic care, patient choice, and the exercise of individual rights.

Apart from the changes in the social context of death and dying, palliative care can also be seen as a response by the health care community to cope with the 'fallout' from life-prolonging medical interventions. Before the advent of modern medicine almost all medical care was palliative in its strictest sense. Now, palliative care generally occurs after a course of curative treatment has been abandoned. This is different to the situation of never having had an expectation of cure, and calls for a different set of attitudes and therapeutic options to offer for the continuing care and comfort of terminally ill people.

This definition of palliative care, which stresses its general approach and philosophy, is not structured enough for the purposes of evaluation. To achieve the goals of the palliative care approach, clinicians need to have a set of interventions and therapies that support and relieve the dying; these can be labelled 'palliative care skills'. Some of these skills are widely practised by non-specialist clinicians, while others require more training and tend to be offered by those who have specialized in the care of the dying and have achieved specialist status; either through accreditation or simply long experience. This section and the next describe the palliative skills which, together, further define the nature of both specialist and non-specialist palliative care.

Expert symptom management

A large part of the impetus behind the setting up of hospices and palliative care teams was the belief that the pain of terminal illness, especially the pain of progressive cancer, can be controlled effectively, and that under standard medical and nursing care too few patients receive adequate symptom control who need it. Relief of physical symptoms is largely the foundation upon which all other aspects of palliative care rest since 'No man can come to terms with his God when every waking moment is taken up with pain or vomiting' (Doyle *et al.* 1993). The focus on pain and symptom control, through a variety of pharmacological and non-pharmacological methods, places much of the clinical practice of palliative care alongside the medical specialties of anaesthesia, medical oncology, and radiotherapy. It would be a mistake to assume that palliative care means low levels of medical intervention—in general it does not. While there may be a reduction in investigative procedures, 'radiotherapy, chemotherapy and surgery all have a place in palliative care provided that the symptomatic benefits of treatment clearly outweigh the disadvantages' (World Health Organization (WHO) Expert Committee 1990).

Expert psychosocial support

Openness in communication, a willingness to listen to the fears and anxieties of patients and their families, and a commitment to support and spend time with patients as they move towards death are characteristics of the palliative care approach. Psychosocial support can mean a variety of things but in palliative care it is conceptualized as the type of care that would be offered by a nurse, doctor, social worker, chaplain, and 'ordinary caring person' all rolled into one. The team approach is thus vital, since no one professional can offer all these types of care at the same time. In addition to these counselling and caring skills, there is also a concern with the practical aspects of terminal care, both for the patient and for the patients' home carers. This can include advice on financial matters (state benefits as well as personal finances), equipment and aids to facilitate home nursing tasks, co-ordination with other sources of statutory and voluntary support (community nurses, volunteers to help with shopping or transport), as well as a 24-hour general advice line.

Forms of care

In what settings are the palliative care skills already described delivered? The specialist palliative care services clearly have no monopoly over caring for terminally ill people and the remarkable diversity in their form which has now emerged reflects the necessity of working alongside mainstream (or conventional or non-specialist) health care professionals in many of the settings where terminal care is provided. Specialists in palliative care thus work in the community, with community nurses and general practitioners (GPs); in acute care hospitals alongside oncologists, general physicians, and surgeons; and in community hospitals as well as nursing homes. In addition, the hospice model of care has continued to flourish (in some countries more than others), with a substantial number of cancer deaths actually occurring in these settings. In some areas in the UK, for example, 12–20 per cent of all cancer deaths occur in independent hospices.

Why evaluate?

Over the past 20 years, dedicated palliative care services in many countries have received considerable charitable funding and voluntary support from the general public. Services have expanded and proliferated on the assumption that 'more' is always better, and have done so in the absence of overall national policy. Local fund-raising has financed some of the setting-up costs of inpatient units and home care teams, while the national cancer charities have pursued their individual agendas in the financing, planning and support of patient services and educational initiatives. Many of the services that were originally instigated by the national cancer charities or developed from local fund-raising have come to depend on funding from the statutory sector. In the UK, formal limited statutory support of the independent hospice sector was given in 1987, with the allocation of funds administered through district health authorities. This was accompanied by the requirement that health authorities should review their palliative care services and plan future developments in partnership with the voluntary sector, with the recommendation that health authority support for hospices should approach the 50 per cent level (NCHSPCS 1994). In 1993/4, the government's special allocation to hospices came to an end, with the expectation that the newly reorganized National Health Service would provide the machinery for the long-term funding of hospices and other specialist palliative care services (Neale *et al.* 1993).

Pressures for the evaluation of specialist palliative care services have been coming from a variety of directions:

(1) from health care commissioning agencies (district health authority purchasers in the UK, health insurance companies in other countries) to ensure that the grants, contracts, and reimbursements awarded to specialist providers (either with or without joint charitable funding) represent good value for money, that the services meet the needs of the population, and that demonstrable 'health gain' is obtained;

(2) from hospital management or clinical directorates within hospitals to ensure that allocating resources to specialist

palliative care teams increases the standards of terminal care within hospital settings;

(3) from specialist palliative care service providers and managers to improve the quality of service delivery and to ensure that patient and home carer preferences are being taken into account;

(4) From the specialist palliative care practitioner to assess the efficacy of new and existing forms of therapy.

Perhaps the greatest interest in palliative care evaluation comes from the health care commissioning authorities—partly because reliance on voluntary support has placed the planning of palliative services outside the direct control and management of the statutory services, but also because with an ageing population and a policy shift of encouraging the transfer of non-acute care into the community, the effectiveness of the palliative care sector is likely to be increasingly important.

Evaluation research strategies in palliative care

This final section of the chapter moves on to discuss the application of evaluation strategies to the field of palliative care. As already discussed (see p. 11), there are principally three research strategies which can be used in evaluation research—experimental (and quasi-experimental), survey, and case study—and these will be briefly examined in turn in relation to the research record. In addition, the use of naturalistic inquiry in palliative care research will be touched upon.

Experimental and quasi-experimental methods Emphasis on the methodological purity and rigour of the randomized controlled experimental design has been a feature of the past 30–40 years of evaluation research. Where randomization is not possible, ethical, or practical, the quasi-experimental design has been recommended as a second best option. The development of statistical modelling techniques and the recognition of the limitations of exercising excessive manipulation and control over situations (which in reality are dynamic and multifaceted) in order to achieve randomization, has brought this wider appreciation of the use of quasi-experimental designs. Contrasting experimental and quasi-experimental methods, a methodological debate centres around the balance between internal and external validity (internal validity refers to the extent to which research findings report a true cause and effect, external validity refers to the extent to which research findings may be generalized to different populations, settings, and types of treatment) and the use of different types of measurement.

One of the criticisms of the randomized controlled experiment (apart from those relating to the difficulty of achieving laboratory-type control in 'field' situations) has been that the findings have not been of widespread relevance either to planners who have to target services at wider patient groups than those commonly included within experiments, or to the individual practitioner when faced with a patient whose background is more complex than the generalized inclusion and exclusion criteria to which trial results refer. Although theoretical refinement to the randomized controlled trial methodology continues as well as developments in the combining of results from different randomized controlled trials through meta-analysis, some advocate the development of a more theory-driven approach which attempts to model the various threats to both internal and external validity in the research. Under this approach, randomization may be used if applicable, but may not necessarily constitute the only safeguard of internal validity, once the threats in a study have been adequately identified and statistically controlled (Chen 1988).

Chen (1988) suggests that the loudest critics of experimental methods of research are those who have faced the most difficulty in attempting to apply the principles to their field of interest. Randomized controlled trials have a rather dismal record in palliative care research. Either they fail to show any substantial difference between control and intervention group (for example, Kane *et al.* 1984; Addington-Hall *et al.* 1992) or they fail for logistical reasons (for example, McWhinney *et al.* 1994). Few randomized controlled trials have been attempted, and those studies which have used quasi-experimental methods have also faced methodological and practical problems (Greer *et al.* 1986; Gray *et al.* 1987; Dunt *et al.* 1989). Rinck *et al.* (1997) provide a useful systematic review of 11 randomized controlled trials undertaken in palliative cancer care, and point out that the methodological problems were so severe in two studies that no results were reported.

Since the early 1980s, commentators on the state of research and evaluation in palliative care have highlighted the following problems in analytic studies (Mount and Scott 1983; Torrens 1985; Kane 1986; Higginson and McCarthy 1989; Goddard 1989 and 1993; Twycross and Dunn 1994, Rinck *et al.* 1997):

(1) lack of sensitive and appropriate outcome measures which reflect 'quality' of palliative care;

(2) challenges to design integrity through incomplete data collection and attrition rates;

(3) lack of refinement of comparative 'units' of analysis, and end-points, and problems with self-selection (lack of patient population homogeneity);

(4) lack of consensus on whose perspective should arbitrate on the quality of care;

(5) difficulty in measuring costs.

Despite these challenges, demands for evidence of effectiveness have not diminished (McQuay and Moore 1994; Ling and Penn 1995), and with the experiences of past research studies to hand, researchers are continuing to attempt to carry out experimental studies and to synthesize the results of controlled clinical trials (Rinck *et al.* 1997).

Survey methods Surveys have been utilized with far more success than experimental methods in palliative care research, and although they cannot examine cause and effect relationships, they have been able to generate a substantial amount of descriptive data. Survey methods have been used particularly to describe service activity (that is, the coverage of palliative care services) and also the prevalence of symptoms and problems amongst patients and home carers. The latter kind of investigation has proved useful in assessing the need for palliative care interventions. Surveys aim to collect standardized information from a specific population group by means of interview or questionnaire, either to produce a 'snap shot' of the state of affairs at one particular time (cross-sectional study), or to monitor change over time (longitudinal research). Surveys in palliative care which have depended upon patient-generated data have faced some of the methodological problems encountered in clinical trials already mentioned, while surveys targeted at the bereaved relatives of patients have their own set of difficulties relating to recall bias and proxy reporting.

Case studies   Again, the case-study approach has been used very widely in palliative care research, and much of the formative evaluation work that has been carried out has tended to focus on particular cases; a hospice, a home care service, a hospital support team, or even an individual patient. It is of course a strategy or approach rather than a distinct method, since it will tend to employ multiple methods of data collection. The point of the case study is however to investigate a phenomenon (the case) in depth and in context. While surveys tend to collect a small amount of information from a large sample of respondents, the case study is concerned with collecting large amounts of information about a small number of 'cases'.

Naturalistic inquiry in palliative care research   Recognition of the limitations of the logical–positivist approach to data collection, particularly to the collection of information about the meaning and impact of social behaviour and action, has stimulated the development and use of more naturalistic approaches. These approaches have the following characteristics: research is carried out in the context or environment of the focus of enquiry (not in the laboratory or at 'arms' length' using a postal questionnaire); the researcher tends to be the data-gathering instrument (using the techniques of observation and interviewing, and recording the outcomes of these); qualitative rather than quantitative data is usually collected; meanings and interpretations are negotiated with respondents, rather than being imposed or deduced; and results will often to be reported like a case study. A range of labels, each with their particular epistemological subtleties, are applied to this sort of inquiry—'post-positivistic', 'ethnographic', 'phenomenological', 'humanistic', and 'hermeneutic', to name a few (Denzin and Lincoln 1994). There are theoretical differences between these approaches, partly because they have developed within different disciplines, although their approach to data collection and analysis are broadly similar.

The ethnographic approach has been successfully used in many areas of health services research. This method was originally used by anthropologists to study the cultural, social, economic, and religious patterns of small-scale societies or well-defined groups within larger societies, using the techniques of participant observation, interviewing, archival research, and community surveys where appropriate

(Bernard 1988). Within health services research a more limited or focused kind of ethnography is often used, which concentrates on a specific area of inquiry (Krefting and Krefting 1991). The research may be carried out principally through interviews and only a limited amount of participant or non-participant observation may be used. Relating back to traditional ethnography however, focused ethnography does attempt to describe the multiplicity of personal, environmental, and organizational factors which impinge upon the subject under study. The approach may in addition employ various other techniques to explore individual and group experiences, for example, diary keeping or other forms of artistic expression, and focus groups (Millward 1995).

The analysis and presentation of qualitative data is governed by the mode of collection and the extent to which theory generation is a major concern. The 'grounded' theory approach of Glaser and Strauss (1967) represents a way of processing and analysing qualitative data in an explicit manner according to certain guidelines, and is now commonly used and referenced. However, the development of theory is not always an end result of qualitative research. All qualitative research is concerned with the generation of concepts which describe, explain, and interpret the field of enquiry, and frequently such conceptualizations remain the major product of the research.

Qualitative approaches are increasingly used in evaluation research because of the need to 'understand complex behaviours, needs, systems and cultures' (Ritchie and Spencer 1994), and there has been an accompanying attention to theoretical and methodological concerns in qualitative data collection, analysis and applicability (Denzin and Lincoln 1994). As well as developing ways to reduce some of the logistical difficulties involved in qualitative research, researchers are also being encouraged to be more explicit in explaining the mechanics of the transition from conceptualization to the emergence of theory (Bryman and Burgess 1994). Fitzpatrick and Boulton (1994) point out that rigorous and transparent attention to qualitative methodology is needed to convince audiences of the value of insights into the 'black box' of health care'—although of course this observation applies equally well to other methodologies.

The strengths of qualitative methods in palliative care research are seen in the flexibility and responsiveness of data collection, and also in their capacity to uncover meanings which are inaccessible using other means (Clark 1997). A concern with the experiences of patients and their carers, their perceptions of and satisfaction with care, and also the meanings which they attach to terminal illness, can all be captured through relatively unstructured dialogue, managed through the one-to-one interview, or even through focus-group discussions.

Conclusion

Evaluation has become an important activity for health care planners and policymakers, as well as service providers. In times of economic retrenchment and fiscal constraint, evidence concerning the effectiveness, efficiency, acceptability, and appropriateness of services is important for resource allocation decisions. Evaluation research is not however a straightforward process, and this chapter has suggested that the link between research and practice is not always as explicit as it might be imagined, and that the prevailing interpretation of evidence-based practice may be inappropriate.

This opening discussion of the nature of evaluation research and how it differs from basic clinical or health services research provides a reference point for the chapters which follow. These chapters take forward many of the methodological issues raised above, and examine first the ways in which patients can be involved in the assessment of palliative care, then how patients' home carers can be used as reliable commentators on the concerns of patients as well as their own satisfaction with the family-centred focus of palliative care. Chapter Four considers how the work of the professional carers can be evaluated, and how the impact of providing care can be assessed. The last two chapters consider the service level effects of palliative care, and suggest a practical framework for future use in palliative care evaluation.

2

Researching people who are terminally ill

Introduction

The aims of specialist palliative care to meet the physical, emotional, and spiritual needs of people who are terminally ill sets an interesting task for evaluation studies in the application of these aims. For example, are patients receiving specialist palliative care better supported during their terminal illness than those not receiving specialist input? Do they have a 'better' death? And what do we mean by a 'good' death, who judges it, and how can we tell whether it has happened?

There are of course many ways to conceptualize a good death. Walter (1994) discusses the theme of the good death and suggests that health care professionals may well hold a different idea of what death should be like than patients themselves; a point supported by others (Johnston and Abraham 1995; Payne *et al.* 1996). Whatever preconceptions are held about what constitutes an ideal death (at peace, pain-free, and so on) what is at issue is whether the activities of the health professional make a difference to the journey through the final moments of life, and the comfort and ease with which death is approached. The task of evaluation is thus to focus on the processes of care that lead up to death, and how these are important in the way in which death is anticipated collectively (that is, what we all think about the way we care for people who are terminally ill), as well as how effective these processes are in the care of individual patients.

In order to evaluate palliative care there have to be clear objectives and associated standards related to the overall aims. This obviously goes beyond mere definition, to a detailed indication of the actual procedures, assessments, and types of care that are provided by specified practitioners, usually within specified time periods. Substantial progress has been made in drawing up general standards of palliative care internationally (for example, WHO guidelines 1990), nationally (for example, Royal College of Physicians 1991), and regionally (for example, in the UK, Trent Hospice Group Palliative Care Core Standards 1992; and in Canada, MacDonald 1993). In addition, many teams continue to establish their own standards or service specifications. However, do the research instruments or techniques exist to evaluate these standards, and how far should 'good palliative care' be separated from the concept of the 'good death'?

It is well accepted in other areas of health care, for example in chronic illness, that patients' perceptions differ markedly from objective evaluations of their health status. Shanks observes, ' A patient who feels ill but is judged healthy by a doctor is not in error and quite correctly rates the outcome as poor; the doctor may be entirely accurate in his or her objective measurements and may have delivered the best possible treatment' (Shanks 1993). In similar vein, Rose writing on the death of a friend from AIDS, observes that 'Even if you are holding his hand, you can never be sure in what spirit your friend has died' (Rose 1995: 110). Quite clearly, how a person judges the care that is provided will depend on factors additional to the actual (objectively assessed) quality of the care, including outlook on life and the extent to which personal goals had been fulfilled. Indeed, Nuland observes that the 'dignity that we seek in dying must be found in the dignity with which we have lived our lives' (Nuland 1997).

This chapter focuses on the issues concerned with researching people who are terminally ill using their perspectives and concerns, and actively involving patients in the collection of data. There is a difference between research that requires patients to actually participate in disclosing information, and research that distils information from the medical, nursing, and social work records, or by clinical observation and judgement. Many clinical trials which have limited outcome measures do little more than approach patients for consent at the beginning of the trial. Thereafter, patients are more or less absent from the research process, with all follow-up data being taken from the clinical records or from blood samples. This chapter examines the former kind of patient-based data, and reviews the range of methods that have been used to engage terminally ill people in the research process, and what drawbacks there are to this.

The difficulties facing the researcher of palliative care can be divided into those which relate to the ethics of palliative care research, those concerning the practical aspects of study design, and those connected to the extent to which study results are useful for evaluation purposes. This chapter considers each area in turn.

Ethics and access

The study of ethics in medical research stresses the balance between the desire of researchers to extend knowledge with the rights of research subjects. Allied to this is the patient's right to autonomy and the doctor's duty to act in the patient's best interests. Does research involving patients who are terminally ill uphold the principle of beneficence which is at the heart of the doctor/patient relationship?

A debate which surfaced in the pages of the journal *Palliative Medicine*, focused on whether research is morally justified with people who are terminally ill. Louise de Raeve asked whether there are 'certain questions that we should never ask', and she framed her question within both a Kantian perspective (that people should not be treated solely as a means to an end) and a risk/benefit perspective (that explores the potential harm that patients might incur while participating in research) (Raeve 1994). Her deliberately provocative article drew fire from a number of eminent palliative care physicians and oncologists who pointed out that Raeve's arguments were generally applicable to all clinical research, not just palliative care, and that her caricature of research as being either paternalistic or unethical was as an unrealistic portrayal of the efforts to base clinical practice on evidence rather than hearsay or instinct (Mount *et al.* 1995).

An extreme position, like that proposed by Raeve, draws attention to the range of factors that should be considered in palliative care research. Few would actually question the need for conducting more research, as long as it is appropriate and well designed (Bruera 1994); so many questions of effectiveness and acceptability are currently unanswered, and for policymakers, the need to plan services on the basis of need relating to effectiveness, cost-effectiveness, and acceptability, is a priority. However, the following points can be highlighted:

1. To safeguard the interests of patients when they are under medical and nursing care, the procedures of asking for and obtaining consent to research should be clearly monitored. Protocols for obtaining consent for clinical trials are relatively well established, although there are still instances when patients refusing to participate have been made to feel isolated (Thornton 1992). With reference to qualitative research methods, apart from Raeve (1994), others have questioned whether consent should not be renegotiated during the course of the research, and indeed, whether consent is a relevant concept for this kind of research. By its nature, qualitative research is exploratory, can be open ended, and in the health care context, can also become quasi-therapeutic (Raudonis 1992; Twycross and Dunn 1994). To ensure that consent is ongoing in a study (during follow-up encounters) it may be advisable to repeat assurances that patients are free to withdraw from the research at any time. However, researchers should also be aware that increasing frailty may affect patients' understanding of ongoing consent.

2. However satisfied researchers feel with the process of obtaining fully informed consent, the impact that the research will have on the patient should be borne in mind. Regardless of the study design, most data collection affects the participant and this needs to be carefully assessed in palliative care research. For this reason, all research work should be piloted in order to ensure the appropriateness of the study instruments or techniques, and to confirm the practicality of the recruitment targets. Qualitative work may well be appropriate at this stage to investigate the burden of the study instruments on the research participants.

3. All palliative care research should be submitted to a research ethics committee. Although such committees are not formal assessors of the research methodology, going through the process of presenting research aims to a critical audience can have the effect of highlighting poor, or impractical design. Seeking ethics committee approval is a requisite for externally funded research projects, and should also be standard for 'in-house' research, during the course of routine care. The temptation to circumvent ethics committees however, often arises from the idiosyncratic and obscure decision-making processes of such committees, rather than from the desire to carry out unscrutinized research. Since this does not serve the wider interests of the research community, the administration of ethics

committees should run in a timely and efficient manner, and alternative arrangements to facilitate the conduct of multicentre studies should be explored (Cartwright and Seale 1990; Clein 1997).

4. Researchers need to be flexible about the completeness of observations and the timing of any follow-up. To ensure that the demands of research do not excessively invade the privacy of terminally ill people, worsening symptoms, including confusion and inability to concentrate, may mean that researchers have to abandon instruments which involve lengthy interview or self-complete questions.

All clinical research needs to be conducted in an ethical manner and these points apply in a general fashion, although in the case of palliative care research they operate with more force because of the physical (and sometimes emotional and cognitive) frailty of the research participants (Bruera 1994; Kristjanson 1994). Since palliative care is most frequently provided for people suffering from cancer, the complex fears and anxieties that accompany a cancer diagnosis are also a factor in the cautious approach. As Bryant and Payne (1993) point out, 'anyone researching into cancer is entering into a very sensitive and complicated area of human concern'. A proportion of people do not like to reflect on their illness experience, nor talk about cancer *per se*, and this of course needs to be respected within a flexible research approach.

There are several ethical aspects in relation to palliative care research. One concerns the vulnerability of the research subjects/participants, as already discussed; another relates to appropriate research design. Given the high vulnerability of the patient population, it is especially important that research which is poorly designed, and unlikely to achieve its objectives, should be discouraged.

The question of whether it is ethical to carry out randomized controlled trials of palliative care (rather than trials of palliative therapy within a palliative care or oncology setting) is a slightly different issue. Trials are only really justified when there is genuine uncertainty regarding the effectiveness of alternative courses of action or treatment. While palliative care clinicians may be convinced of the benefits to be brought by palliative care in general, they may be uncertain as for whom it works best, at what time, and in which setting. However, policymakers may want an answer to the general question of whether palliative care services are a good investment or not, and may not be content with the assertions of palliative care practitioners that they do deliver high-quality, effective care. The pressure to prove the benefits of palliative care necessitates patient-based research, and given the safeguards already discussed, researchers can seek to minimize any adverse effects of research. Setting such activities within a context of quality assurance and needs' assessment may make the research effort something which patients and their families can accept.

Measured outcomes

Quality in palliative care can be summed up in words and pictures, but health care commissioners, managers and planners generally prefer numbers; numbers indicating the percentage population who have received an effective service, and numbers indicating pounds or dollars that represent an efficient spend of the health care budget. This chapter now moves on to consider the ways in which information derived from patients can describe or 'measure' the palliative care they receive. The first section considers measurable outcome indicators, and the second, the findings from qualitative research.

The past 10 years have seen an emerging recognition that patient perceptions of their quality of life and their care or treatment preferences need to be taken into account in clinical research. It is not sufficient to measure the outcomes of treatments only in terms of mortality, morbidity, and survival rates; an assessment of their social and psychological impact upon patients is also necessary. Acknowledging the multidimensionality of health care outcomes and devising ways of measuring them has become a major field of inquiry within the health sciences, not only within cancer research but for all clinical specialties. Two separate strands in this research have recently converged: one is the continued development of health status measures; and the other is the interest in quality of life measures. For a time, as Brooks (1995) describes, these two fields of interest ran parallel, but latterly, it has been clear how much they have in common. Both stress the importance of measuring physical, psychological, social, emotional, and spiritual dimensions to obtain a fuller picture of either what it means to be 'healthy' in general terms, or what 'quality of life' means to people who are undergoing various medical treatments. The psychometric issues involved in questionnaire development and validation are of course the same for both sets of measures (Streiner and Norman 1989). Health status measures have generally been developed and tested within general populations and their applicability to subsections of populations, for example, people with cancer, or terminally ill people is not established. On the other hand, considerable work has been carried out to develop quality of life measures for patients with cancer, and various assessment tools are available specifically for use in the palliative care context.

The intention of this section is not to review the various quality of life instruments in detail. This has been done very adequately elsewhere: for cancer generally (Bowling 1995), palliative oncology (Girling *et al.* 1994; Montazeri *et al.* 1996*a* and *b*; King *et al.* 1997), and for palliative care (Clinch and Schipper 1993; Finlay and Dunlop 1994). Instead, this section will examine some of the concepts behind quality of life measurement, and also the issues which need to be borne in mind by researchers wanting to use quality of life measures for palliative care research. The focus of this section is therefore on structured measures, while the next section discusses the use of less structured means of eliciting patient concerns and perceptions.

The quality of life concept

Clinical trials and surveys largely depend on the measurement, and sometimes rating, of a wide range of patient based characteristics. These may be grouped conveniently into four main areas: socio-economic and demographic factors (age, occupation); biomedical factors (co-morbidity, biological response, biochemical markers, survival); health service utilization factors (length of hospital admissions, frequency of visits to the doctor, estimates of direct medical costs); and quality of life factors (psychological and spiritual dimensions, patient perceptions of severity of symptoms and their burden). There is a distinction between measures that are taken to describe the characteristics of the patient (the first three), and measures which seek to represent the patient's sense of well-being. It is now widely accepted that the success of clinical interventions needs to be assessed by both descriptive measures and measures that attempt to record patients' perceptions of how they feel, in order to provide clinicians with the widest sense of the effect of different treatment regimens. This is particularly so in palliative care, where the main aim is not to achieve a cure or postpone death, but to improve the comfort of patients in their final months, weeks, and days (Richards and Ramirez 1997).

Quality of life is thus a major concern in palliative care, although its definition is notoriously problematic. Despite the observation from many that ultimately 'satisfactory quality of life is an individual judgement' (Finlay and Dunlop 1994) and that its meaning 'is dependent on the user of the term, his or her understanding of it, and his or her position and agenda in the social and political structure' (Bowling 1995), its measurement has been vigorously pursued, notwithstanding the apparent inability to conceptualize it. Researchers in the health field are relatively content to work within a theoretical framework of *health-related* quality of life— a subconcept of global quality of life. Restricting what is included in health-related quality of life still results in an impressive array of domains: physical function, emotional and psychological function, social function, role function, spirituality, and treatment satisfaction are some of the main areas identified as being important to assess.

Quality of life measures can be divided into those which are (a) generic, (b) disease specific, (c) diagnosis- or cancer site-specific, (d) domain specific, and (e) treatment specific. The tremendous range of measures that have been developed, many of which overlap with each other, means that selection of the most relevant and sensitive (able to detect change) measures is most important within the research context.

Generic scales are those which include questions on a number of the domains taken to be important in quality of life, and which are used with different populations (and disease groups). These include measures such as the Nottingham Health Profile (Hunt *et al.* 1981), the SF (Short Form) -36 (Ware and Sherbourne 1992), and the General Health Questionnaire (Goldberg 1988). Disease-specific questionnaires in this context refer to the multidimensional scales developed for use with cancer patients, such as the Rotterdam Symptom Checklist (de Haes *et al.* 1990), the European Organization for Research in the Treatment of Cancer (EORTC) quality of life core questionnaire (Aaronson *et al.* 1993), and the Functional Living Index—Cancer (Schipper *et al.* 1984)—to name only a few. There can be an overlap between some of these questionnaires and others which concentrate on general and specific symptoms such as the McCorkle's Symptom Distress Scale (McCorkle and Young 1978). Domain-specific measures are those which concentrate on a particular aspect of quality of life such as anxiety and depression (Zigmond and Snaith 1983), pain (Melzack 1987), coping (Folkman and Lazarus 1988), mood (McNair *et al.* 1992) and depression (Zung 1965). (See Bowling 1995, for an overview of scales relating to psychological morbidity.)

Site-specific questionnaires have been designed to elucidate some of the problems associated with particular cancer sites, which may not be adequately picked up in general symptom scales. The development of site-specific modules for the EORTC questionnaire (see previous reference), and site-specific extensions of the Multidimensional Quality of Life Scale—Cancer (Padilla *et al.* 1992) reflect this concern. For example, patients with head and neck cancer tend to have a different set of anxieties and problems relating to eating, communication, and breathing than, for example, patients with colorectal cancer who may have their own set of anxieties concerning bowel habits and coping with a colostomy. Likewise, a small number of questionnaires have been developed which are specific to certain sorts of treatment such as chemotherapy for patients with breast cancer (Levine *et al.*, 1988 cited in Bowling 1995) and for those having undergone bone marrow transplantation (Grant *et al.* 1992, cited in Bowling 1995).

All of these scales are self-report, and during the course of a study, may be completed on several occasions. The first set of responses would constitute the baseline measurements against which subsequent responses would be compared. The timing of questionnaires and completeness of response to all items is thus a matter of importance in the extent to which the results become useful. Some studies use batteries of instruments to collect global quality of life measurements, as well as detailed domain-specific or site-specific information. While these may be accepted by patients in clinical trials in oncology, who will be able to complete them during outpatient clinic visits or inpatient admissions, patients who are terminally ill with advanced cancer may not tolerate long or multiple questionnaires. There is also the question of whether such scales are actually appropriate for assessing the goals of palliative care.

Using quality of life measures in palliative care research

Quality of life measures can be used in at least three possible ways in palliative care research:

1. They can be used in surveys of palliative care populations for descriptive purposes. The subscales which are included in some of the measures are able to provide estimates of the occurrence of depression, anxiety, pain, and so on, which can also be used in assessing the need for various services or targeted interventions.

2. The measures can be developed and used as an aid to clinical decision making and managed care. For example, some measures may have an emphasis on functional ability to help inform assessment of the needs of the individual patient (Kaasa *et al.* 1997).

3. Within clinical trials, quality of life measures are used as indicators of the quality and effectiveness of clinical care (outcome measures). It is hypothesized that changes in quality of life may reflect the type of medical and non-medical care received.

However quality of life measures are used in practice, there are a range of design and conceptual issues which are highly pertinent to their value in palliative care research. These issues are now examined in some detail.

Design issues

While the conceptual validity of quality of life and symptom report instruments is of concern (and discussed below), questions over their administration are also important.

Mode of completion of questionnaires   Much of the attention of research in palliative care is focused towards the few months or weeks before death, which is when many patients are referred to specialist palliative care services, particularly inpatient hospices. Because such patients are often referred with uncontrolled symptoms and other distress, a variety of techniques have been used to elicit information. Some researchers have utilized self-complete quality of life or symptom report questionnaires, while others have depended upon observer-rated questionnaires completed by professional staff or family carers. The 1990s has seen considerable work in the development and refinement of self-complete quality of life instruments for use with palliative care populations. Much of this work is an extension of the quality of life instruments initially designed for cancer populations in the oncology setting.

Peruselli *et al.* (1993) used an Italian version of the self-report Symptom Distress Scale with a group of 43 patients being monitored at home by a pain therapy and palliative care division. The patients completed the questionnaire within 48 hours of beginning home care, and at least once a week thereafter. Only patients who had completed two or more questionnaires were included in the analysis (data are not given as to how many patients failed to complete two questionnaires). The authors found that the analysis of the average weekly score was an effective way of identifying symptom distress variations, and they concluded that using the total score offered a partial assessment of the efficacy of home-based palliative care (Peruselli *et al.* 1993).

Ventafridda *et al.* (1990) report the use of a self-complete questionnaire in their cross-sectional study of quality of life during a palliative care programme (although the methodology states that completion could occur with assistance from a relative). No information is actually provided relating to the validity and reliability of the questionnaire; the authors suggest however that the results demonstrated the capacity of the palliative care programme to enhance the quality of the lives of terminally ill patients.

A number of other questionnaires are currently under development and psychometric testing at the time of writing. The McGill Quality of Life Questionnaire is being developed by clinicians and researchers in Canada, specifically for people with advanced cancer (Cohen *et al.* 1995). Following its testing in eight palliative care services, it has undergone revision, but its authors claim that the instrument can be used to compare the quality of life of different groups of patients (Cohen *et al.* 1997). Sterkenburg and Woodward (1996) report the development of another scale for palliative care populations. The McMaster Quality of Life Scale has 32 items covering four dimensions of quality of life: physical, social, emotional, and spiritual. To date, testing of the scale appears to have been carried out on a relatively small population (84 patients), and further work is reported to be continuing with refining the instrument (Sterkenburg and Woodward 1996). A further scale under development is the Hospice Quality of Life Index, which as its name suggests, has been developed particularly for use in the hospice setting (McMillan 1996). Again, the scale has been tested on a relatively small population of 118 patients enrolled in two American 'not-for-profit' hospice programmes.

Other self-complete questionnaires are more clearly oriented toward diagnosis and assessment rather then the measurement of quality of life. The Edmonton Symptom Assessment System (Bruera and MacDonald 1993) is a self-complete assessment tool which consists of nine visual analogue scales (including pain, shortness of breath, nausea, depression, activity, well being, drowsiness, and appetite). The developers report good compliance amongst cognitively aware patients, and they recommend the scale as an effective test for baseline and subsequent assessment of symptoms. MacAdam and Smith's (1987) assessment of suffering questionnaire was developed primarily as a needs' evaluation technique, and went beyond other measures at the time in attempting to accommodate the perceptions of patients who were terminally ill. Rathbone *et al.* (1994) have taken this concept one step further and devised a self-evaluated assessment schedule for use with hospice patients. This consists of a mixture of staff and patient-centred assessments, with the intention of using one set of assessments to complement the other. In their study of this tool, the authors found that 58 per cent of the 55 patients who took part in the study identified problems not recognized by the medical or nursing staff, with the majority of the problems being of a psychosocial nature. Ellershaw *et al.* (1995) report the development and use of the PACA (Palliative Care Assessment) tool by the King's College Hospital (London) advisory palliative care team. It is considered to be easy to complete and enables the palliative care team to obtain a rapid overview of the main problems of each patient.

Much of the symptom-based research work that has been carried out amongst patients receiving specialist palliative care has tended to rely on visual analogue scales for the reporting of intensity of symptoms. For example, the evaluation by Griffith *et al.* (1990) of the palatability of Oramorph used seven visual analogue scales relating to taste preference; Johnson and Miller's (1994) study of the efficacy of choline magnesium trisalicylate in the management of metastatic bone pain utilized visual analogue scales to construct a pain intensity difference score; and Lynch *et al.* (1992) employed both visual analogue and verbal rating scales to assess pain in their study of the role of intrathecal neurolysis for perianal and perineal pain. While visual analogue scales (VAS) appear to be easy and quick to use, they have been criticized on a number of counts; in particular, they present difficulties to patients who are unable to mark the VAS line with a pen, and some patients have difficulty relating their experience to the extreme states which form the anchor points (Choinière and Amsel 1996).

Many other studies have relied on observer assessments, using functional status measures such as the Karnofsky or Eastern Co-operative Oncology Group (ECOG) scales (Karnofsky and Burchenal 1949; Zubrod *et al.* 1960) and quality of life scales such as Spitzer's Quality of Life (Spitzer *et al.* 1981). Similarly, many of the assessment tools developed for use specifically in the specialist palliative care setting rely primarily on completion by staff or other observers, for example, the STAS (Support Team Assessment Scale) measure (Higginson 1993*a*), the Edmonton Functional Assessment Tool (Kaasa *et al.* 1997), and the San Diego Severity Index (Strause *et al.* 1993). In addition, there are a number of observer-rated scales which assess functional ability and dependency of patients for the purpose of determining likely workload within the palliative care setting (Williams 1995; Anderson *et al.* 1996).

The use of self-complete questionnaires is not always straight-forward in a population of people who are terminally ill. For such measurements to be meaningful, completion of the questionnaires has to be timely and entire, and patient groups need to be well defined. The practical and methodological difficulties encountered in the design of studies which depend on structured questionnaires, as well as the problems of interpreting the results are now discussed.

Sampling   In general, sampling procedures vary according to (a) the intervention or process being studied; (b) the setting in which it is delivered; (c) the time period over which the study will take place; and (d) the research method being used. Because this chapter is concerned with patient-based research, sampling here is discussed in relation to prospective studies (trials and longitudinal studies) and cross-sectional studies. Retrospective studies are discussed in other chapters.

There are two main problems relating to sampling in palliative care research. One is determining the sampling frame, or the population from which to draw the sample; the second is recruiting sufficient numbers of patients to meet the statistical power of analytic studies (Faithfull 1996). Practically, palliative care research can be broken down into two levels for evaluation purposes:

(1) Evaluations of the effectiveness of specific palliative therapies within specific settings, such as analgesia administration, models of counselling support, or liaison protocols between primary health care teams and specialist providers;

(2) Evaluations of the effectiveness of different models of palliative care provision, such as inpatient hospice care and hospice at home care, or specialist care and standard mainstream care.

Evaluations carried out at the service level are likely to consist of a number of subevaluations of the different components that make up the service, in as far as they can be analytically distinguished and measured. The relationship between these subevaluations and the overall evaluation may be assumed to be unambiguous, although in practice it is likely to be problematic, since the efficacy of individual therapies may not in itself provide evidence of the effectiveness of palliative care as a system of care.

To evaluate the effectiveness of individual therapies, having a relatively limited indication for their use and a reasonably narrowly defined outcome, the randomized controlled trial will be the best method to use, although as Calman and Hanks observe 'the nature of palliative medicine practice means that the number of patients who may be suitable for entry to a particular study will be small . . . Most drug studies will involve inpatient observation . . . patients who are stable enough to be considered for such studies will rarely want to remain as inpatients in the palliative care unit or hospice' (Calman and Hanks 1993). Multicentre trials and *n*-of-1 trials have been suggested as ways of retaining the experimental method in such evaluations, while overcoming problems of patient recruitment. Multicentre trials are common in the evaluation of new cancer drugs; their logistical complexity, expense, and robustness are well discussed in Pocock (1983). The *n*-of-1 trial (Guyatt *et al.* 1990) may be of relevance to palliative care research, but the potential length of follow-up, together with the confounding effect of newly arising clinical problems associated with the disease progression, may limit its use in far advanced disease. The *n*-of-1 trial may be a better patient-based approach for people who are relatively stable in their symptoms, and who are not imminently terminally ill, although Sackett (2 June 1995; personal communication) suggests ways of introducing a 'bail out' for periods in which patients are faring poorly, and going on to the next stage of treatment. This shortens the trial and provides another outcome measurement: time on treatment. Exploration of this methodology is required in palliative care research; *n*-of-1 trials may prove to be a robust method of assessment in the future, and would thereby circumvent the recruitment difficulty of narrowly defined explanatory clinical trials, as well as provide clinicians with 'confidence in their management decisions' (Guyatt *et al.* 1990).

Experimental and quasi-experimental models of research have been applied to questions of palliative care *service* effectiveness. Underlying the practical and conceptual problems with such studies is the assumption that people do not refer themselves, or get themselves referred, to hospice services completely randomly. Policymakers wish to plan services on the basis of population need, yet specialist palliative care services may be a form of care that some people feel they can take or leave. There is an element of 'electiveness' about palliative care, involving a considerable measure of patient preference, that implies that the concept of clinical indications for palliative care may not apply universally. It is unknown what proportion of the population with terminal illness would wish to be cared for by specialist palliative care services, at which point during their terminal illness, and at what level of input (just the symptom control or the range of psychosocial interventions as well). It is also unknown how many people who would appreciate and need specialist palliative care input have access to the services, and what proportion do not. Equally, it is unknown how many people who do receive specialist palliative care services actually benefit from them.[1]

An associated uncertainty is whether people who do wish to use the full range of palliative care services are systematically different in their health service utilization patterns, their attitude towards

[1] An inclusive approach to palliative care needs' assessment has been developed by Higginson (1997), for use in the UK context

terminal illness and death, and their families' capacity to cope with bereavement than people who do not. In which case, there are conceptual problems in deciding the sampling frame of evaluative studies. Is it methodologically more accurate to take the general population of terminally ill people to be the sampling frame, or is it sufficient to take only those patients actually referred to palliative care services and deny some of them the benefits of specialist palliative care input? In the former case a comparison would be made between people receiving a specialist service, and those not, in the assumption that in all other respects they are matched—possibly a false assumption. In the latter case, people would be matched in terms of their inclination to accept specialist input, but the results would not be generalizable to the wider population (Vainio 1993).

Prognosis Following on from the difficulties in establishing a sampling frame, are the questions of prognosis and comparative end-points. Generally in health care research, comparable patient populations are identified through measures of interval from a critical incident (for example, point of diagnosis, organ failure, or surgical procedure) or by illness severity indicators. In palliative care research, there is a difficulty in identifying when palliative care input is appropriate and how far it can and should overlap with curative and aggressive treatment, and debate over whether it is vital to have comparable groups in terms of likely survival time *and* symptom severity *and* psychological adjustment in order to assess the effect of palliative care. Current debate over the boundaries of palliative care suggest its appropriateness in some form from the time of cancer diagnosis, as well as being applicable to patients with other clearly defined terminal illnesses (progressive neurological conditions) and those with less apparent terminal illnesses (stroke, chronic obstructive airways disease).

For the purposes of palliative care research, two methods of assessing prognosis have been used: clinical judgement (observation and judgement based on experience); and structured prognostic indicators (for example, Rosenthal *et al.* 1993). The accuracy of both methods varies according to the length of prognosis which is given (that is, one year, six months, three months, or a final few days) and also the number of times applied to individual patients. As Maltoni *et al.* observe (1994) clinical observations generally overestimate survival times, particularly in the final six months, and also have a large measure of inaccuracy when applied to prognoses of about one year. Various performance status scores have been used to predict life expectancy, among them the Karnofsky or ECOG scale (Karnofsky and Burchenal 1949; Zubrod *et al.* 1960), as well as the presence or absence of certain symptoms. In reviewing these measures, Maltoni *et al.* concluded that although a low performance score appears to be strongly correlated with imminent death, a high score may not predict long survival (Maltoni *et al.* 1994). Quality of life measures (such as Spitzer's Quality of Life scale) have also been used for predicting likely prognosis, but with inconclusive results; suggesting that they can be used with more accuracy at advanced rather than earlier stages of terminal illness (Tamburini *et al.* 1996; see also den Daas 1995 for a review of the literature relating to length of survival in end-stage cancer). Maltoni *et al.* suggest that the way forward may be in developing a multidimensional prognostic index linked to biological and nutritional factors, and performance status and symptoms—not only for the purposes of research, but to facilitate the planning of treatments and care packages (Maltoni *et al.* 1994).

Because of the difficulty of identifying comparable patient groups from the outset, the answer can be to collect detailed follow-up information on patients until death, and then retrospectively form comparable groups working back from the point of death. This was the method used by the National Hospice Study (Mor 1988) and also by Hinton (1994) in his reported prospective study of patients being cared for by a hospice home care service. It raises questions over the size of study needed for statistical purposes, and whether a study is lengthened (to an unknown degree) by waiting for all patients eventually to die or instead recruits large numbers of patients initially in order to accrue enough finished care episodes within a shorter study period (since outcomes are generally assessed in relation to proximity to death). Either research strategy has implications for resources and management, and for the way in which follow-up assessments are carried out.

The importance of comparative end-points varies according to the research question. In some situations, evaluations may focus on the process of referral to a palliative care service, and will concentrate on factors that are independent of likely prognosis or illness severity. However, where there is considerable variation in the total length of time spent under a palliative care service, differences in prognosis may become an important confounding factor.

Contamination and confounding   Specialist palliative care is rarely provided without the backdrop of other supportive services offered by health and social care professionals. Also, in some situations patients may experience specialist palliative care from different teams in different settings. For example, in the UK, a patient may be admitted to hospital and referred to the hospital palliative care team; discharged to the community where the primary health care team takes over, asking for specialist advice from the community based palliative care team; and finally admitted for terminal care to the local hospice. Would an experimental method of assessing the effectiveness of the hospital palliative care team preclude patients in the placebo or control arm of the study from seeking community palliative care input or hospice care? And how can the results be interpreted if it were known that the non-specialist community nurse of a 'control' patient had recently completed a course in palliative care?

In addition to the unknown quality of medical, nursing, and social care provided by mainstream professionals, patients receive very different levels and intensities of specialist service. For example, a study recently carried out by the author and colleagues, showed that the services received by a district-based population of patients who died in 1993 and had been referred to the hospice located in the district included the following: inpatient care, day care, advisory home nursing care (from the hospice programme itself), as well as care offered by liaison nurses in the acute care hospitals. Out of a total of 1384 people who died with cancer given as either a main or underlying cause on their death certificate, 659 (48 per cent) had been referred to hospice services. The combinations of different service inputs are shown in Fig. 2.1. In addition, 91 (14 per cent) of this referred subgroup also received day care services at the hospice. Although we found that over 70 per cent of the patients received home care nursing input, variation in the length of time between referral to the service and death ranged from under a week to over two years. For patients who died within one year of referral, the median length of time between referral and death was eight weeks (mean = 12, mode = 1). The number of visits received was also highly variable. For 28 patients, referral came too late for any

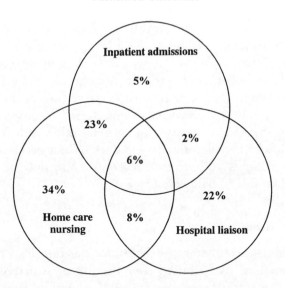

Fig. 2.1 Types of hospice service offered to people who died during 1993
in one health district

visit to be made, and in the remainder, the number of visits ranged
between 1 and 106 (mean = 7.4, median = 5, mode = 1). On the basis
of these results, calculating the sample size of a cohort or quasi-
experimental prospective study would need to take into account the
statistical power required to carry out subgroup analyses caused by
these kinds of variations.

Confounding is a major threat to the validity of any analytic
study. In palliative care, in particular, it is an extremely important
source of difficulty in interpreting data. Confounding factors include
those related to diagnosis and personality, as well as the perception of pain and other symptoms, and ways of coping. Much of
the palliative care research in hospices is carried out in the general
assumption that people with advanced cancer share the same kinds
of needs for palliative care. For example, Maltoni (1994) states that
'data from different studies seem to confirm that, after a certain
stage, the natural history of tumours assumes a common pathway
in which the presence of particular symptoms does not correlate
directly with the primary site of the disease' (Maltoni 1994).
Contrary to this assertion, an international cross-sectional survey,
looking at pooled data on 1840 cancer patients from seven palliative

care centres, showed that the prevalence of symptoms does differ to a significant degree according to the primary site of cancer (Vainio *et al.* 1996). Some studies do present their data by primary cancer site but the numbers per site are usually too small to make statistically meaningful comparisons. However, given the fact that people with certain cancers tend to be referred to hospice services more than others, it is unclear how generalizable such results are, and indeed, whether the primary site does have a pervasive impact on cancer patients' differential response, not only to curative treatment but also to palliative care.

Conceptual issues

Even in the absence of some of the difficulties just described, there are still questions to be raised over the use of structured health-related quality of life outcome measures; questions and concerns which have been acknowledged by numerous researchers over recent years. It is encouraging that there is ongoing refinement of the instruments and continuing conceptualization of the issue of 'quality' in palliative care. A discussion of these areas of development is briefly presented.

Sensitive and relevant instruments   Many researchers have pointed out the difficulties of obtaining answers from frail patients, and questionnaires have been simplified and shortened in order to place less of a burden on such patients. Finlay and Dunlop recommend for example that self-complete questionnaires in the hospice setting should not take more than 15 minutes to complete (Finlay and Dunlop 1994). While shortening questionnaires and reducing the total number in the 'battery' is important, researchers have also tried to improve the simplicity of data capture. For example, Choinière and Amsel (1996) discuss the use of a visual analogue thermometer (a sort of slide-rule-type instrument for patients who have difficulty using a pen), while Gaston-Johansson (1996) reports the development of the 'Pain-O-Meter' (a pain assessment tool made of plastic, with slider, for measuring and describing pain using a visual analogue scale and the choice of 11 affective word descriptors).

   It has been observed that the symptom lists which are part of many of the frequently used quality of life scales, are often too comprehensive, with the result that the overall assessment is liable to become viewed, by the respondent, as irrelevant or inappropriate. A different approach is therefore now tending to be taken, employing various instruments that have space for patient-volunteered problems and concerns. The McGill Quality of Life Questionnaire (Cohen *et al.* 1995) and the PACA (Palliative Care Assessment) tool (Ellershaw *et al.* 1995) both begin by eliciting the most troublesome symptoms from the patient, and then measuring the burden of these symptoms, rather than presenting a list of symptoms, many of which might not be applicable (see also Rathbone *et al.* 1994). In the McMaster Quality of Life Scale (Sterkenburg and Woodward 1996) respondents can check a 'does not apply' box against the lists of symptoms, so reducing the number of symptoms that they are required to rate. Other researchers have taken this approach further, developing a scale (the Schedule for the Evaluation of Individual Quality of Life or SEIQoL) based entirely upon volunteered problems and concerns which are related to self-evaluated quality of life (Hickey *et al.* 1996). Using this approach, patients are first asked to volunteer five areas of concern which are important to their quality of life, and then to rate the current performance of these areas against a 10 cm visual analogue scale. Finally, they assign weights to each area, according to the priority each has for them in relation to the other areas. This direct weighting method uses five interlocking coloured discs (a colour for each area of patient concern). The discs are presented to the patient who is asked to move each one in relation to the others so that each non-overlapping area corresponds to the relative importance of the concern represented by that segment. It is then possible to derive a quality of life index by computationally combining the VAS score with the weighting score. The authors report the use of this method with a cohort of individuals with HIV and AIDS. However, it has also been used with palliative care populations, and the methodology has been developed to include volunteered symptoms as well as quality of life concerns (D. Waldron, personal communication).

How far these patient-generated measures can be used for comparative purposes is not yet clear. However, the potential use of this kind of approach for research purposes should be explored, particularly as it parallels other methodological developments in patient-generated outcome research in other areas of clinical care (Coulter 1991; Ruta *et al.* 1994). It is important that patients should feel that the research instruments are sensitive to their own concerns, and indeed that they can control aspects of the type and content of information transfer.

The meaning of quality of life scores in the palliative care setting
Many of the instruments just described have been developed for use in the oncology setting with cancer patients, and some have shortened versions for ease of use in the palliative care setting. There is a question whether generic cancer questionnaires are relevant to palliative care; the goals of the latter are more diverse than those of anticancer therapy (Richards and Ramirez 1997). A question remains as to the value of quality of life scores as outcome indicators of palliative care service quality—how significant are they?

Selby suggests that quality of life is now established as an outcome measure, a prognostic variable, an aid to patient management, and a target for therapy in clinical cancer research (Selby 1993). Others are not so confident in the progress so far in examining the meaning of quality of life scores. Lydick and Epstein (1993) question whether, in terms of the individual management of patients, results that are statistically significant are also clinically significant. They also wonder about the relevance of such results at the population level. Lydick and Epstein attempted to catalogue the various ways in which quality of life researchers have operationally defined clinical significance or meaningfulness, and found that they separated into two broad categories: one they termed distribution-based (based on the statistical distributions of the results); and the other, anchor-based (where changes in quality of life measured were anchored to other clinical changes or results). They recommended that statistical significance should not be confused with clinical significance and that more attention should be given to the development of methodologies to express quality of life changes in meaningful terms, at both the clinical and public health level (Lydick and Epstein 1993).

An interesting example which illustrates this uncertainty is the report by Addington-Hall *et al.* of the findings from their randomized controlled trial of a co-ordinating service for terminally ill cancer patients (Addington-Hall *et al.* 1992; Raftery *et al.* 1996). In the first report (1992) the authors reported few differences between the intervention and control groups in terms of quality of life (Spitzer's Quality of Life Scale) and other variables. However, the later report (1996) of the economic evaluation that was carried out alongside the trial reveals statistically significant differences in costs between the two arms of the study—the co-ordination service was more cost-effective than standard services. Although this study was not evaluating the impact of a palliative care service itself, many aspects of the co-ordination service are similar to those typically provided by some palliative care providers. What is interesting is that quality of life data did not seem to reflect differences between the groups, yet cost data (an arguably 'harder' type of outcome) did.

Whether quality of life data are able to measure the effect of the input of palliative care depends on the domains which are measured, and what sort of input is likely to impinge on those domains. While this is rather an obvious point to make, it is also interesting how increasing amounts of research are producing more sophisticated understandings of these various domains of life. To conclude this section, a short discussion of some of this research is presented.

Domains of life important in quality of life: deeper understandings
The control of pain and other physical symptoms has been taken to be central to the contribution of palliative care, and that is why there is an emphasis on measuring these areas. Considerable work has been carried out in the area of pain which reveals how complicated and multifaceted the pain experience is, and consequently how difficult it is to assess comprehensively. Structured instruments appear to go from the sublime to the ridiculous; either asking a few questions ('Do you have pain?', 'How severe is the pain?') or asking tens of questions to obtain a detailed description of its source, location, frequency, effectiveness of relief, and so on. Detailed questioning can however result in fascinating information. A survey of 111 patients with advanced cancer and pain who were newly referred to a palliative care centre found that patients reported 370 pains (a median of 3 per patient) (Twycross *et al.* 1996). Forty per cent of the patients experienced four or more pains, while cancer accounted for 46 per cent of the pains. The results of this survey have a number of implications for the clinical management and assessment of patients with pain, but the results also suggest that the answers to short questions about pain in quality of life questionnaires have to be treated with some caution. Indeed, a full assessment of pain may require attention to its intensity, functional capacity of the patient, mood and personality, pain beliefs and coping strategies, information about medication, as well as psychosocial history (Jamison 1996).

The psychosocial care offered by palliative care services is also difficult to assess; partly due to a lack of definition and conceptualization of the various components of this area of care, and also due to a shortage of baseline information concerning what changes might reasonably be expected in a population of advanced cancer patients receiving palliative care. The need for more research on this subject has already been highlighted (Vachon *et al.* 1995). Psychosocial care may be separated into a number of different areas, for example, social, psychological and spiritual support. Recent work on social support has attempted to apply some aspects of this area by measuring the size, density, and composition of patients' social networks, as well as the degree of perceived emotional and instrumental support (Courtens *et al.* 1996). Psychological support is more difficult to assess. The use of various instruments to measure psychological morbidity, for example the HADS (Hospital Anxiety and Depression Scale) (Zigmond and Snaith 1983), have been used for screening purposes and prevalence studies but it is unclear whether they are an appropriate outcome measure of a specific kind of psychosocial intervention (apart from, presumably, appropriate medication) (Grassi *et al.* 1996). While spirituality may not strictly be included with psychosocial issues, there is an overlap in questions relating to guilt, anxiety, fearfulness, and so on (Dudley *et al.* 1995; Cawley 1997). Assessing spirituality, and the extent to which spiritual concerns are elicited and addressed within research studies is still at a rather problematic stage, although Millison (1995) provides a review of some of the scales which have been used to measure the spiritual needs of patients.

Attempting to refine and extend the concept of quality of life for patients with advanced cancer receiving palliative care will no doubt continue to be a matter of considerable interest (for example, see Rustøen's (1995) plea to include 'hope' with quality of life) and rigorous psychometric testing. However, as an introduction to the next section it is interesting to note that after apparently several years of developing and testing a quality of life instrument, a number of researchers state that 'MQOL [McGill Quality of Life] scores or scores on any questionnaire will never replace the richness of a face to face, in-depth conversation . . . The QOL gold standard for individual subject evaluation in this patient population may thus entail qualitative methodology, an approach which may more readily plumb the depths of individual subjective well-being' (Cohen *et al.* 1997).

Qualitative assessment of patient concerns

The demands of analytic research methods for measurable outcomes and quantitative representation of patient perceptions of symptoms and concerns can lead to frustration with the inflexible, closed, and structured nature of this approach. The goals of palliative care to alleviate physical, psychological, and spiritual distress mean that the assessment of patients referred to palliative care services has to be multidisciplinary and multidimensional. This approach acknowledges the uniqueness of each patient and attempts to tailor the care package to the patient's needs, rather than fit the patient into a rigid framework of care options. Such variability in meeting patients' needs is a potent source of confounding in experimental studies (as discussed earlier). At the same time however, it is regarded as a strength and a quality indicator of palliative care. Since palliative care does not consist of a narrow range of therapeutic procedures which, when applied, have the same effect in each patient, to attempt to quantify and describe operationally what it is in practice— including the manner in which it is delivered, received, perceived, and judged—is surely a Sisyphean task. But accepting that clinical care has to be assessed for its integrity and appropriateness, it must be strategic to consider the use of assessment methods which can better cope with the range of patient- and situation-based variables which clinicians and researchers know, from personal and anecdotal experience, affect individual quality of life.

As an alternative to self-complete measures, patient concerns may be elicited through means of interviewing; either relatively structured to obtain responses to a number of predetermined topics, or fairly unstructured, to allow patients to express their concerns and opinions with minimal prompting and probing. Both forms of investigation have been used in the palliative care setting, as well as structured observations of the care of patients. In addition, case studies may be used as a method of reporting individual examples of care; not usually with the intention of drawing generalizable conclusions, but as a means of illustration. The use of these different qualitative methods are now described in relation to (a) the meaning and perception of illness; (b) patient satisfaction and preference; and (c) processes of care.

Qualitative methods require a different kind of approach than quantitative methods. The investigator, as the data collection 'tool', is important in relation to what information is elicited and how, and whether, (s)he can manage the interview process in a way that leaves both informant and interviewer intact. Asking patients about hopes and fears, expectations and anxieties can be distressing if not controlled within an appropriate framework. Just as doctors and nurses require a particular set of communication skills for caring for people who are terminally ill, so too do researchers. Balancing the researcher role with other potential roles can be difficult. There is the possibility, raised by de Raeve (1994) that some forms of qualitative work become quasi-therapeutic, and this can bring both dangers and opportunities. Lichter *et al.* (1993) describe the use of a technique called 'life review' with hospice patients who are considered to feel that their lives appear to lack meaning. Through the construction of a biography with a trained volunteer (non-counsellor) patients find that recounting their life story brings satisfaction and an understanding of their individuality (Lichter *et al.* 1993). While biography is presented as therapy in this case, the telling of life stories can be an important part of qualitative research, especially when a rapport is being struck between informant and interviewer; a life story can be presented as the context in which patients' experiences can be understood. There are no hard and fast rules about carrying out qualitative research, however every researcher needs to be aware of the boundary between research and counselling/caring, and have a system of recognizing and dealing with the processes of entry into and exit from other peoples' lives. Threats to the interests and sensitivities of the informants, and to the validity of the data collection process, have to be minimized. Because such work frequently raises questions about how well researchers are dealing with the data collection, and how competently they manage their role, the work has to be set within a project management system, with support available for the researchers from project team members.

The meaning and perception of illness

Explorations of the beliefs terminally ill people hold about their illness and symptoms commonly uncover a multidimensional and multilayered web of meaning. Ferrell *et al.* (1993) explored the meaning of pain to patients with advanced cancer under the care of home health care agencies in California by interviewing 10 patient–

care giver–nurse triads. The authors describe how three categories of meanings of pain emerged: (1) immediate causes (related to the cancer illness); (2) the social and personal effects of the immediate causes; and (3) ultimate causes. They remark that the number of responses in which subjects mentioned or implied the influence of God on the pain experiences was high enough to question the need for future study, encompassing the effect of cultural/religious diversity on the experience of pain, and identifying appropriate interventions.

Given the interest in structured quality of life measures, some researchers have asked patients what quality of life actually means to them. Berterö and Ek, for example, describe the meaning of quality of life to adults with acute leukaemia, and reveal how it is given meaning on different levels, with a positive outlook being its superior dimension, interpersonal relationships and autonomy constituting the next level of importance, and then security, support, respect, information, and conversation being the next important set of qualities (Berterö and Ek 1993). Tigges (1993) criticizes hospices for concentrating on superficial symptoms as markers of quality of life and not attending to the nature of human beings and how enhanced quality of life is realised. From his research, he suggests that loss of quality of life is caused by feelings of helplessness (loss of control), hopelessness (inability to see any purpose in living), and uselessness (no perceived personal worth or value).

This kind of work describes the immensely diverse meanings that are attributed to various states, which also co-exist and interact with cognitive impairment (Bruera 1994), clinical depression, and other conditions, some of which may respond to pharmacological and non-pharmacological types of treatment. Researchers suggest that it is important for clinicians to uncover the meaning of quality of life that individuals hold, relative to their own lives, and hence the ways in which each may best be helped. Some might argue that this is best done within a phenomenological approach (for example, Gullickson's (1993) use of Heidegger's notion of the authentic and inauthentic self as a way of locating the various meanings held about death), others may argue for a grounded theory approach (for example Kagawa-Singer's (1993) study of models of health among patients with cancer), while yet others may eschew theory application or building for the insights of individual patient profiles or vignettes. However, whatever the methods of uncovering patients' meanings, this kind of approach assumes that palliative care staff know what to do with the knowledge when they obtain it. Not all staff can cope with other peoples' existential crises, and it is a matter of sensitivity to realize what patients should be encouraged to reveal for good therapeutic purpose, and what should remain a matter of personal responsibility.

Patient satisfaction and preferences

Assessing patient satisfaction with palliative care services is a different question to assessing the effectiveness of palliative care, but nonetheless it is a central concept in evaluation. Field's (1994) review of client satisfaction with terminal care summarizes many of the methodological and practical difficulties of this kind of research, which apply as much to experimental methods and surveys as they do to forms of naturalistic inquiry. Broad assessments of service satisfaction are not generally very informative, although narrowing questions down to specific issues can be more fruitful. Considerable attention has focused on the use of patient surrogates (home care givers and staff) in the assessment of the adequacy of care and where preferences for location and types of care were achieved. (Home care givers as patient surrogates is discussed in the next chapter.)

Qualitative approaches have been used to explore patient satisfaction with the amount of information given about diagnosis, prognosis, treatment options, and so on. In palliative care, openness in communication and providing informed options for patients is regarded as an underlying principle, although the way in which communication is managed may well vary from culture to culture. Coughlan's (1993) study of knowledge of diagnosis amongst a group of 30 patients receiving chemotherapy for cancer in Ireland revealed that most (26) knew their diagnosis. This contrasts with Centeno-Cortés' study in Spain of 97 patients with advanced malignant diseases (33 patients admitted to the palliative care unit, and 64 to oncology services) in which only 32 per cent (31) had actually been informed of their diagnosis. Interestingly the authors found that 42 per cent of the patients admitted to the palliative care unit had been informed, compared to 27 per cent of those admitted to the standard oncology service. This study suggested that communication with the patients was better in the palliative care unit, although the level of disclosure overall was rather low (Centeno-Cortés and Núñez-Olarte 1994).

Preference for place of death is an important theme running through the questions of service planning in palliative care, and was an issue investigated by Townsend *et al.* in their 1987 study using structured interviewing techniques to elicit patient opinions. This study revealed however, that not all patients can express a preference, and that preferences change during the course of terminal illness (Townsend *et al.* 1990). This finding was supported and refined more recently by Hinton (1994).

Processes of care

Another important contribution of qualitative methods to evaluation research lies in its focus on the situation and context in which care is delivered. It is not always enough to record what people say (whether through questionnaires or interviews); observation of the manner in which care is delivered and the kind of routines and practices which surround it is also needed. The ethnographic approach involves the structured observation of care encounters and interactions between patients, patients and staff, and staff, all of which are important in the care environment, whether it be in the hospice, the nursing home or on the hospital ward. Hockey's ethnographic comparison of death and dying in a residential home and hospice stands as an important example of the strengths of this method. Although her findings are not directly generalizable to all residential homes and hospices, through her use of various literary techniques, she provides a sense of what it might be like to be a client in these settings, thus sensitizing the reader to a range of issues seldom raised (Hockey 1990).

Many of the naturalistic or ethnographic studies which have been carried out have focused on staff perspectives on the caring process and these will be discussed in Chapter 4. However, Raudonis' study (1993) took the perspective of the patient and attempted to describe the impact of empathic nurse / patient relationships on patient outcomes. Fourteen terminally ill adults receiving home hospice care were recruited for this study, and each patient was interviewed using open-ended introductory questions. Since empathy has been identified as a major component of relationships in nursing and related disciplines, the focus of the study was on how far patients identified their relationships with the home hospice nurses to be based on empathy, what form this took, and how it affected them. For the 10 patients who described experiencing an empathic relationship with their nurses, this was felt to be achieved through the latter acknowledging the former's personhood—that is, through offering friendship and being willing to spend time getting to know them, approaching them as 'people with an illness' not 'ill people', and by being willing to reciprocate by sharing feelings and experiences. Raudonis defined outcomes in terms of patients' reports of improvements in both physical and emotional well-being, such as one patient's statement that 'she's given me a new outlook and one of not despair. You know, one of hope, of well-being. I don't know how to describe it any more than that, except that she's there' (Raudonis 1993).

Observational studies of quality of life in institutions are important for describing complex social relationships and intricate patterns of interaction. They can reveal more about the atmosphere of an institution than by simply relying on patient, staff, or visitor reports. They are not necessarily straightforward to carry out (Clark and Bowling 1990), nor are they without their ethical dilemmas (Mills *et al.* 1994), yet they can highlight examples of good practice and areas of concern. When undertaking service evaluation, it is possible that such observational methods can be sufficiently sensitive to discriminate between different care settings in a way that survey methods may be unable to do on their own.

Conclusion

This chapter has discussed the range of structured quantitative measures that seek to record patients' problems and sense of well-being, and also qualitative methods of portraying the intricacies of personal outlook. It is important to incorporate patient-based assessments in the evaluation of palliative care, and yet it is clear that there are difficulties in achieving this. These may be practical and ethical, surrounding the design and conduct of prospective studies, while sampling and confounding problems affect the interpretation and meaning of the results.

At present there are no 'gold standard' measures of quality of life for palliative care. A number of self-rating quality of life measures developed for use with cancer patients in the oncology setting are being used in the palliative care setting, and a number of new scales are currently undergoing psychometric testing for use with palliative care populations. Many instruments depend on assessment by staff, and sometimes by home carers. Progress has been made in the area of symptom and functional ability assessment schedules, and their use for monitoring the aims of palliative care with regard to symptom control is certainly well accepted. The extent to which these can be used as outcome measures to compare populations receiving different forms of care is as yet to be established. A new and developing area is in the use of patient-volunteered symptoms (getting the patient to say what is bothering them). The comparison of symptom prevalence measured by these means as opposed to the estimates derived from the more closed, symptom check-list instruments, will be a source of interest in the future.

Qualitative research methods are resource intensive on a large scale, while their local findings may well not be generalizable to other settings. They also produce a wealth of detailed data which, while insightful, may not be focused enough to draw the categorical conclusions which are needed for planning purposes. Yet they are able to reflect the complexity of care in a way that is not possible by other methods, and can also locate the 'caring encounter' within a meaningful context. In relation to palliative care, naturalistic inquiry with patients can reveal the different ways in which they respond to and cope with pain, thus commenting on the construct validity of the structured instruments, as well as describing the organizational context of palliative care delivery.

3
Home and family carers

Introduction

There is a general acceptance that meeting the needs of patients with advanced and incurable disease has to include recognition and support of the needs of the family members and friends who are the patients' primary, non-professional carers. Caring for the carers is important in terms of (a) their own preventive health care; (b) maximizing care options for the patient; (c) facilitating current health policy towards increased community based care; and (d) enhancing the quality of patient care by focusing on family dynamics and the home caring context. Accepting that the needs of home carers come within the legitimate remit of palliative care services, the question can be asked as to what indicators linked to home carer well-being and satisfaction can be used in evaluation studies of palliative care. This chapter considers these issues, and explores the various methodologies which have been used to investigate the impact of caring on home carers, as well as the extent to which the views of home carers may be taken to be representative of patients' views. To begin, however, it is important to establish what is meant by home carer, how many people with terminal illness have home carers, and what are the demographic characteristics of this population.

The literature abounds with different terms to describe the people who look after other people, who may be slightly or considerably more dependent and incapacitated than themselves. Because carers do not necessarily live under the same roof or may not be related to the dependent person, the generic term 'family carers' is not always technically correct—12 per cent may not be co-resident (Addington-Hall *et al.* 1991), and three to six per cent are friends and neighbours (Jones *et al.* 1993; Wakefield and Ashby, 1993). 'Lay carers', 'home care givers', 'informal carers', 'unpaid carers', 'family care givers' are terms that have all been used instead to refer to those people who are identified as a primary non-professional carer, although of course, many people who become terminally ill do not have someone close enough to them to become a primary carer. (The figure may range from 18 per cent (Yang and Kirschling 1992) to 27 per cent (Addington-Hall *et al.* 1991) for people unable to identify a primary helper or carer at home.) In this chapter, the phrase 'home carer' will be preferred, as a term broadly indicating the source of care from the domestic/private/informal domain, and will be used as shorthand to include related and non-related, co-resident and non-co-resident carers.

Home carers of people terminally ill with cancer have been found to have a different demographic profile to home carers generally (Seale 1989). Because the average age of people dying from cancer is younger than that of people dying from other causes, the average age of their home carers is younger, they are more likely to have sources of care and support within the home, and thus the possibility of spreading the burden of care amongst more people (Neale 1991). Various studies have examined the characteristics of the home carers of people with advanced cancer with the following general con-clusions. Between 48 and 66 per cent of home carers are spouses, with possibly two-thirds being wives (Jones *et al.* 1993; Wakefield and Ashby 1993; Addington-Hall *et al.* 1991), while around 20 per cent are likely to be daughters (or daughters-in-law). Overall, around 66–75 per cent of all primary home carers of people terminally ill with cancer are female (Jones *et al.* 1993; Yang and Kirschling 1992; Given *et al.* 1993); a higher figure than the 60 per cent previously quoted (Neale 1991). Just under half of all home carers are less than 60, and only a very small proportion (around four per cent) are likely to be aged over 80. The prevalence of disability or chronic illness amongst carers prior to their caring role, or which develops during the process of care has not been widely investigated, although various studies have described sleep problems and loss of weight amongst carers (Jones *et al.* 1993). Some families may have prior experience of cancer amongst their members, and indeed, some carers of patients terminally ill with cancer, may themselves have been diagnosed as having the disease, at some point in the past or at the same time as the patient.

These age and gender features of carers suggest that picking up the pieces from terminal cancer illness is likely to be a concern for widows and middle-aged daughters primarily, although the pattern of cancer illness itself drives a characteristic path through certain

sorts of families. An early death from breast cancer often involves
families with young and teenage children; childhood leukaemia involves younger parents and grandparents; while the caring involved
in terminal illness from prostate cancer may fall predominantly upon
an elderly wife. Just as the type of cancer affects the needs and
concerns of the sufferer, so it also reflects the stage in the family life
cycle of the home carers. Problems of confounding, in studies of
patients terminally ill with cancer, due to different cancer sites is
also likely to be replicated in studies of their home carers. Carers
are clearly not a homogeneous group; they vary according to the
demographic characteristics already discussed, their interpretation of
their caring role (Finch and Mason 1993), their personalities and
capacity to cope, and their socio-economic status.

As Smith and Regnard imply in their flow diagram of managing
family problems in advanced disease (1993), families are not always
a haven of moral or practical support. Many families are characterized by what some might label dysfunctional relationships,
resulting in barriers to communication within the family and
between the family and health care professionals, and difficulties
in coping with the crisis brought on by the terminal illness. But
equally, many families do not automatically have problems with
coping with terminal illness in one of its members, and indeed,
coping with the stresses of caring can ebb and flow. Measuring the
impact of terminal care on home carers, both in the weeks leading up
to death and afterwards, is not a simple task for all these reasons.
Clark suggests that there are four areas of concern relating to
research into informal care (1993*b*). The first is with the identification of informal carers and their definition, the second is with the
meaning that surrounds the caring role for the individuals concerned, the third is with the need to evaluate palliative care services
by taking separate account of the perspectives of the carer and
patient, and the final area of concern is with the constant need to
ensure that all research is carried out after full ethical review and
approval, with the consent of the participants, and with due regard
for the sensitivities of all those involved. Both Neale's (1991) and
Clark's (1993*b*) reviews of informal care are good starting points for
the interested reader.

This chapter takes the perspective of the home carer and looks at
various ways in which he or she has become the focus of study in
palliative care research. Much of this work is descriptive, although a

significant strand is the use of various indicators to analyse the effect of different models of care on subsequent adjustment during bereavement, and satisfaction with care.

Impact of terminal care on carers' well-being

Various studies have calculated that people who are terminally ill with cancer spend as much as 90 per cent of their time at home during their illness. Home is usually where people want to be when they are ill. As one terminally ill patient stated, whom Moore interviewed in her study of patients with amyotrophic lateral sclerosis, 'I can watch television at three in the morning, eat at midnight . . . watch my children play baseball . . . I can refuse a treatment . . . have a beer or order a pizza. In other words, be in control' (Moore 1993). Home also appears to be the place in which the majority of terminally ill patients would wish to die, although as Hinton (1994) has shown, carers of those patients admitted to a hospice for the last few days of terminal care still considered that the patients had had home deaths because that is where they had been cared for predominantly. Clearly, a home death does not always have to mean actually dying at home. Home is also where government policy in many countries now wishes patients to be, for convalescent and rehabilitation purposes, as well as terminal care. However, for this lucky convergence of sentiment regarding home-based care to work properly, there has to be easily accessible inpatient facilities for respite care (Griffith 1993); provision for when complications to the illness require urgent intensive medical or nursing interventions; and also the offer of terminal care, when either patient or carer (or both) feel that home is no longer an appropriate place to be. As importantly, there have to be sufficient community based resources to provide a level of clinical care, support, and respite for the home carers to enable the patient to be adequately cared for at home.

There is a wide literature on the effect of caring on people's lives. The financial costs, the emotional and psychological costs, the costs of social and employment opportunities foregone, and the unremitting nature of everyday reality as a carer have been vividly described (Glendinning 1992; Jones and Peters 1992; Ross *et al.* 1993). Much of this work relates to carers of people with illnesses associated with advancing age, such as arthritis, senile dementia, circulatory problems, and other disabilities or special needs. People with these problems may not be imminently terminally ill, and the expectation of length of care can be very open ended. In this respect, caring for someone with advanced cancer may be different. The caring is more likely to be of an intense and relatively short-lived nature in some cancers, and much more extended in other cases (Seale 1991). In one study, the duration of care giving for 55 home carers ranged from 1–180 months, with an average of 23.1 months and a median of 9 months (Yang and Kirschling 1992).

In general, the literature on the effects of care giving suggests a range of negative responses to caring such as anxiety, exhaustion, stress, strain, health-related problems, financial hardship, and role conflict; while the positive responses include a sense of challenge, finding more purpose in life, and achieving family closeness (Herth 1993). Yang and Kirschling (1992) present an excellent short review of the literature on caring, and from it propose three main outcomes of caring: amount of lifestyle change, care giver role strain, and rewards of care giving. The question which they investigated in detail through their study of 55 care givers is whether the length of time under hospice care and duration of caring affected these care giving outcomes. The outcome measures used were derived from the scales of Archbold and Stewart, and Montgomery and Borgatta (both cited in Yang and Kirschling 1992), and showed that the sample experienced low to moderate amounts of role strain, a moderate amount of lifestyle change, and a great deal of reward from care giving. The interaction of these outcomes with the duration of care giving and the length of time of hospice involvement were not statistically significant. However, the study revealed—not surprisingly—that when care givers had to deal with behavioural problems in the patient (often arising from impaired cognitive functioning) such as paranoia, suspiciousness, or aggressiveness, this produced increased stress and uncertainty in the care givers.

The extent to which the mental state of the patient affects the mental state of the home carer has also been the focus of research. Given *et al.* (1993) reviewed a number of studies in the area and concluded that even after controlling for prior psychological state, illness events do affect patients' later psychological states and also the well-being or depression of their care givers and immediate families. The study by Given *et al.* (1993) attempted to disaggregate the effect of the different components within the care giving situation, by looking at various factors such as patient depression, patient immobility, physical symptoms, patient dependencies, and care giver optimism with a sample of 196 patient–care giver dyads recruited through six community-based cancer treatment centres in the US. They found basically that patient depression was more associated with the effect of physical discomfort brought on by symptoms and treatment, than with the loss of mobility *per se*. Carer depression was more directly linked with patient lack of mobility and high dependency, and only indirectly linked with symptomatology through the depression felt by patients on account of their physical discomfort. The refinement by Given *et al.* (1993) of earlier work is interesting since it looks at both direct and indirect paths linking patients' physical health with care givers' reactions, and suggests that measures of care giver depression should stand alongside other measures of patient dependency and symptomatology. This finding has been supported by other studies (Speer *et al.* 1995; Kristjanson *et al.* 1996).

The view of home carers

Home carers have a set of needs relating to care interventions which can make their job an easier one, as well as a set of opinions as to how well the health and social services are meeting the needs of their terminally ill relatives. As Kristjanson (1989) observes 'As participants, recipients and observers of care, family members evaluate the care received by the patient and themselves'. Conceptually, it is not always easy to separate out satisfaction with services from satisfaction with the way the various carer and patient roles are being exercised, and the myriad of coping and adjustment mechanisms used by all family members facing the anticipated loss. The family can be viewed as a system, with differing capacities for the care of a member according to the life cycle stage through which it is passing (Jenkins 1989; Smith 1990). It is against this picture of heterogeneity that surveys of home carer satisfaction and needs' assessment are carried out, and these will be discussed.

Studies looking at the needs of home carers and their satisfaction with services can be divided into those which are basically descriptive and carried out for the purpose of local needs' assessment, and those which are more ambitious in their intent and inform the development of structured instruments for use in clinical trials and surveys, and also for audit purposes.

Descriptive accounts can be as circumscribed as the reporting of case studies or personal views. For example, in 1983, the *Lancet* published a widow's account of caring for her 43-year-old neuro-psychologist husband who died of leukaemia, vividly picking out those aspects of care which helped and those which did not; 'Helplessness was certainly a constant emotion. The long wait for platelets, blood, or just a word with a doctor . . . waits which made me feel like a prisoner', and interestingly she observes that during the terminal illness she did not have the time or inclination to ask herself 'how is this affecting me?' or 'what do I feel about this?'. She reports that at first she felt bewilderment, mingled with an understanding of the increasing bouts of illness that led up to the diagnosis, and then an overwhelming desire to change places with her husband, almost feeling it easier to face death than to watch someone else die (Anonymous 1983). Personal cases cannot be used for generalizations—they are emotional and subjective—but they do have a power of description that sensitizes readers to the range of feelings that can accompany caring for loved ones who are terminally ill.

While retaining some of the intimate nature of the personal account, case studies are utilized in qualitative research to con-textualize subjective accounts, and also to allow limited interpreta-tion. A collection of case studies may uncover recurring themes and suggest hypotheses to be further examined. Being very similar to the clinical case study, it is an approach which could perhaps be used to more effect in palliative care research than currently. In relation to exploring some of the concerns of home carers, a study by Mah and Johnston (1993) illustrates the way case studies can be used. The authors collected information about four patient-carer dyads (patients with head and neck cancer) through semi-structured interviews, observations, and chart reviews, over three time periods (before treatment, during treatment, and during rehabilitation). The authors found that concerns varied across the three time periods but were grouped around five categories of cancer and its meaning, social relations, hospital experience, treatment, and future place-ment. They also found that concerns varied between patients and their family carers. To facilitate case-study-type analysis of home carer concerns, Richards *et al.* (1993) recommend the use of geno-grams as a psychosocial assessment tool in the hospice setting. They have found that drawing diagrams of the family structure helps to expose relationships between family members, life cycle issues, and the importance of supportive neighbours, friends, and community resources. The authors point out that the genogram, as a map of the family's contextual systems, can be used by all professionals within the multidisciplinary team.

Qualitative research methods clearly have their place in studies of home carer concerns, but much of the work that has been done in this area has been survey based, using relatively structured ques-tionnaires. Many of the descriptive surveys of home carers have been retrospective; recruiting random samples of bereaved carers usually during the first four to twelve months following the death. A number of these carried out in the UK have broadly followed the methodology of Cartwright and Seale (1990) which has been described in detail in their book *The natural history of a survey*. In essence, this has involved using death certificate returns to form the sampling frame for the survey, and conducting interviewer-administered structured questionnaires with the nearest carers of the deceased sample population, six to twelve months following bereavement. Cartwright pioneered this methodology in the late 1960s, with the first cross-sectional survey of life before death carried out in 1969. In the 1980s she sought to repeat this study, interviewing the nearest carer of a random sample of 639 deceased in England. Various research groups have conducted other studies with interview schedules based on the 'life before death' model—most notably the regional studies of Addington-Hall and McCarthy (1995) from University College, London, and the work of Field *et al.* in Leicester and elsewhere (1992).

The strengths of this method are that detailed information can be collected on the circumstances surrounding a death from the point of view of someone who had been close to the deceased person, providing evaluations of the adequacy of symptom control and the response of the health and social services, as well as identifying carers' needs during terminal illness. Also, the sample drawn is more likely to be representative of the general population since the sample frame is not determined by health service utilization (that is, hospice or hospital use). It is also claimed that this method is able to achieve more detailed and comprehensive information about the

circumstances in the last weeks before death than is possible pros-
pectively, from patients themselves, since many become unable and
unwilling to answer long questionnaires. The weaknesses of this
method, in relation to the extent to which carers can accurately
report the feelings of patients, will be discussed.

Retrospective studies of this nature can again be divided into those
which aim to compare specialist palliative care services with mainstream, standard care, and those which aim to describe the satisfaction with care delivered within specific settings.

One of the objectives of the 1987/8 life before death study of
Cartwright and Seale (1990) was to assess the influence of the
hospice movement on the nature and availability of care, and the
attitudes and expectations of lay and professional carers. Since
this survey took a random sample of all deaths, the number of
people who had received hospice care was relatively low: just under
three per cent died in hospices while another four per cent received
some form of hospice care. The study found that hospice patients
were more likely to know that they were dying than other patients
terminally ill with cancer, and respondents felt that the quality of
both inpatient and home hospice care was better than conventional
care.

Wakefield and Ashby (1993) undertook a survey of attitudes to
terminal care among 100 surviving relatives of people who had died
of cancer in South Australia. They achieved a lower response rate
than Cartwright and Seale (56 per cent as opposed to 80 per cent),
perhaps because they recruited respondents by letter (and follow-up
by telephone in some cases) while Cartwright and Seale recruited
'cold' through unannounced visits by the interviewers. They found
that relatives expressed greatest satisfaction with hospice care in the
cases of death occurring in institutional settings (hospital, hospice,
nursing home, and private hospital). Access to doctors, good
communication, and 24-hour backup of equipment and services
were aspects of care which relatives felt were important (Wakefield
and Ashby 1993).

A study from the US also sought to compare the quality of
hospice care with conventional care by examining the extent to
which basic emotional needs of families were met during a relative's
terminal illness. The study compared relatives of three groups of
patients all of whom died in hospital and were under the care of
(1) a community-based hospice programme without an inpatient

unit; (2) a hospital-based hospice programme without an inpatient unit; or (3) a conventional care hospital. All these groups were compared with each other and with a sample of families whose terminally ill members died at home under the care of a community-based hospice. One hundred bereaved home carers completed a postal questionnaire which consisted of a demographic data form, the Need Satisfaction Scale, the Nurse Satisfaction Scale, and the Overall Satisfaction Scale (Dawson 1991). Statistical analysis of the results demonstrated that the hospice groups scored more favourably on all measures of satisfaction compared to the conventional care group, with the differences in scores being highest between the home hospice group and the conventional care group. Linking the meeting of emotional needs with levels of satisfaction with care proved to be the mechanism whereby hospice care was perceived as being of higher quality; 'families coping with a member's terminal illness have basic emotional needs, the satisfaction of which may influence feelings of satisfaction with the program of care' (Dawson 1991).

Other studies have not sought to make a comparison between specialist and conventional care for terminal cancer illness, generally because of the limited nature of the study. Addington-Hall *et al.* (1991) studied the needs of 80 carers of people who had been admitted to hospitals in an inner-London health district and found that although many patients had received excellent care, there were areas of dissatisfaction including inadequate symptom control, the undesirable nature of dying on busy acute wards, difficulties in obtaining information, and lack of adequate community services and out-of-hours support. Sykes *et al.* (1992) examined the attitudes of 106 carers of people who died of cancer in Pontefract Health District (before inpatient specialist palliative care services were established) using semi-structured interviews, and found that the highest number of adverse comments regarding terminal care arose over the subject of information. This study also drew attention to the fact that carers' experiences at the time of death colour their assessment of all the service received during the terminal illness. In addition, it uncovered instances of inadequate pain relief and lack of information about financial support. Jones *et al.* (1993) collected information from 207 carers of patients who had died of cancer at home in Devon, and found fewer instances of uncontrolled pain than in previous studies (for example, Parkes 1978). The authors concluded that improved pain relief was being provided by primary care teams, augmented in a few cases by specialist nurses, although control of other symptoms (for example, nausea, dyspnoea, and vomiting) was poorer. The major area requiring attention was lack of information about financial benefits and sources of help outside the health service.

A study which looked at the needs of 40 relatives of cancer patients admitted to a specialist palliative care inpatient unit in Scotland, however, produced some surprising results given the findings of Dawson (1991) already described. The study was carried out using standardized scales (28-item general health questionnaire (Goldberg and Williams 1988), a shortened version of the Bereavement Index (Jacobs *et al.* 1986)) in combination with specially designed measures which covered the relationship of primary care givers and patients and the availability of and satisfaction with social support, and included a demographic data form and a 14-item questionnaire designed to measure the nature of care givers needs and the type and frequency of support offered by unit staff. One of the main findings was that care givers who had wished for but not received support from the unit staff reported heightened feelings of anxiety and grief, although care givers who frequently received such support did not indicate less distress or better health than those who seldom or never received help (Pottinger 1991). The author concluded that support by hospice staff may not sufficiently alleviate the distress of grieving relatives before bereavement, while lack of hospice support, if desired (in 15 per cent of care givers), seemed also to cause extra distress to family members. The study of Field *et al.* (1992) of the care and information received by lay carers of terminally ill patients at the Leicestershire Hospice, also suggested that carers may not be receiving as much contact with staff as they could, given the goals of staff to meet the psychosocial needs of the carers as well as the patients. Carers however remained highly satisfied with the care given to the patients. The discussion of Kristjanson *et al.* (1996) of the role of fulfilment theory and discrepancy theory in explaining variance in family care satisfaction is useful. She suggests that satisfaction may be determined by the difference between what a person expects, and what she or he perceives has been given. If expectations in general are inflated, then obviously it will take more effort to produce a perception of satisfaction than if lower expectations were held in the first place.

Authors of some of the studies already described suggest that their findings might be built into standard methods of assessing the needs of home carers (Sykes *et al.* 1992; Pottinger 1991), having identified that routine assessment could have a valuable role. Kristjanson (1989) describes the development of a scale to measure family satisfaction with advanced cancer care (the FAMCARE Scale). This was developed in Canada, through qualitative research with 20 families of patients with advanced cancer in the hospice setting, to identify health care provider behaviours that were perceived as helpful or unhelpful. The next stage of the study used a Q-Sort procedure with a convenience sample of 210 family members to identify those items that were considered more important in the care of the patient and family (Kristjanson 1989). The final phase of development, reported in 1993, was a pilot study to test the validity and reliability of a 20-item scale derived from the Q-Sort with a convenience sample of 30 family members. Whilst she notes limitations of the pilot study due to the small size of the sample and the fact that it was derived from an oncology outpatient department rather than a hospice, Kristjanson concludes that the results suggest that the scale shows potential as a reliable and valid tool to measure family satisfaction with advanced cancer care, although it requires testing with larger groups of patients. In particular, from her results three findings need further examination: (1) that college education is associated with more satisfaction with care; (2) that white family members are more satisfied with care than non-white family members; and (3) that family members of older patients are more satisfied than family members of younger patients (Kristjanson 1993). It will be interesting to see how useful this scale is found to be in the future. Kristjanson *et al.* (1996) report using it in a follow-up study of 80 family members on first assessment (before the patient's death), and 64 family members at three months' postbereavement, with good reliability and validity. Jarvis *et al.* (1996) also used an adaptation of the scale in their evaluation of a palliative care programme, although the size of the sample was low (n = 34) which limits the conclusions which can usefully be drawn from the study. (Kristjanson (1993), provides an interesting review of the literature relating to measurement of satisfaction in the health care setting.)

A scale which has been tested and found wanting in the hospice setting is the Paloutzian and Ellison Spiritual Well-being Scale. In 1989, Kirschling and Pittman reported the results of a study designed to test the reliability and validity of this scale with 70 family members caring for a terminally ill relative. The scale was developed with college students and consists of religious and existential well-being subscales. Although the scale was found to have a high degree of internal consistency and reliability, its construct validity was questionable from comments offered by respondents during the interviews. For example, it could not adequately reflect the feeling that painful, negative experiences can provide the greatest opportunity for personal growth which can subsequently be viewed as positive. Just as quality of life measures with patients have not always managed to pick up the changes in personal growth and spirituality that can occur in the face of progressive physical decline, it seems that such changes in home carers are also difficult to measure.

Although not a scale as such, the questionnaire developed by Cartwright and Seale (1990) and further refined by Addington-Hall *et al.* (1995) is increasingly being used as a method of assessing home carer needs. A question that relates to all these structured methods of assessment is however, to what extent do home carers comment on their own feelings and how far do they reflect the concerns of the patient?

Home carers and patients: do they tell the same story?

Because research with patients who are terminally ill is difficult for practical, ethical, and methodological reasons, the people closest to them have been viewed as patient surrogates or proxies. Asking the home carer how the patient is, what their problems are, and what bothers the patient the most is useful in terms of corroborating patient reports, as well as being potentially the only source of information when the patient is unable to help. To what extent, however, do home carer accounts reflect the concerns of patients, and if they do differ, how important is this?

To an extent, the account of terminal illness and death and the feelings attached, constitute a story made up and rehearsed by the home carers, the patient before death, and also the health care professionals in contact with the family before and after death. Collusion, denial, guilt, blame, unfinished business, sadness, disappointment, and confusion are all factors which may affect the way in which situations are interpreted and the importance given to physical symptoms. How far both home carers and patient are able to report objectively on the experience of terminal illness is difficult to tell and it is possible that a lack of congruence in patient and carer accounts may reflect different versions of the 'story' rather than different degrees of accuracy or sensitivity in observation. Examining the extent to which home carers' accounts can be used as proxies for patients' accounts has become an issue in palliative care research, partly because of the concern which some researchers feel over whether terminally ill patients should be subject to research or not.

Table 3.1 lists a selection of the different permutations of patient / home carer / staff carer perspectives that have been examined in the context of patient surrogacy. These studies broadly show a congruence between home carer and patient perspectives over the presence or absence of relatively clear-cut symptoms and problems. When home carers' and patients' accounts from the time during terminal illness are compared, home carers tend to report higher levels of patient anxiety and distress than patients themselves. When home carers' accounts after the death are compared to patients' accounts recorded earlier, it is suggested that perceptions by the former of symptoms and problems have become more polarized. From her work on this issue, Higginson suggests that changes occur during the bereavement period and family members alter their assessment of the severity of problems, possibly due to the natural processes of grief and coping and changes in mood during bereavement, and possibly due to recall bias (Higginson *et al.* 1994). The agreement between staff, home carer, and patient perspectives is not clear-cut either. Higginson's (1993) study compared staff with home carer and patient perspectives and found that staff members recorded pain as less severe than patient or family member, that patients rated their own anxiety as much less extreme than either team or family member, and that family members perceived more problems than either staff or patient. Staff assessments usually lay between that of patients and family members. Hinton (1996) looked at the reliability of relatives' retrospective reports of terminal illness in relation to their own reports and those of patients given before death. Before death, patients' and carers' reports showed good agreement, but relatives' retrospective reports at three months postbereavement indicate less agreement, particularly in relation to pain, anorexia, and depression (Hinton 1996).

Table 3.1 Congruence between different patient / carer / staff dyads in relation to the severity of patient problems

Comparison	Authors	Sample size	Measures used
Patient with home carer (Before death)	Higginson *et al.* (1990)	65 patient / carer dyads	8 items of care
	Butters *et al.* (1993)	8 patient / carer dyads	9 STAS items
	Spiller and Alexander (1993)	18 patient / carer dyads	10 physical problems, 11 emotional reactions, HAD Scale, preferred place of death
	Field *et al.* (1995)	28 patient / carer dyads	Institute for Health Care Studies questionnaire
	Hinton (1996)	77 patient / carer dyads	Patient / carer volunteered symptoms, rated by 4-point scale
Patient with home carer (After death)	Cartwright and Seale (1990)	34 patient / carer dyads	Symptoms and satisfaction with services (questionnaire developed by Higginson)
	Hinton (1996)	71 patient / carer dyads	Patient / carer volunteered symptoms, rated by 4-point scale
Patient with staff carer (Before death)	Butters *et al.* (1993)	19 patient / staff dyads	9 STAS items
	Higginson and McCarthy (1993)	84 patient / staff dyads	7 STAS items
Home carer with home carer (Before death) (After death)	Hinton (1996)	71 home carers	Home carer volunteered symptoms, rated by 4-point scale
	Higginson *et al.* (1994)	7 home carers	7 STAS items
Home carer with staff carer (Before death) (Before death)	Higginson and McCarthy (1993)	67 home carer / staff dyads	7 STAS items
Home carer with staff carer (After death) (Before death)	Higginson *et al.* (1994)	35 home carer / staff dyads	7 STAS items

Key: HAD = Hospital Anxiety and Depression; STAS = Support Team Assessment Schedule

---

Main findings

Family members rated symptoms and anxieties as more severe than did patients, while they were more satisfied with services than patients.
Small sample size limits conclusions.

Main differences found relating to emotional reactions and state of patients. Home carers more likely to report patient anxiety than patients themselves.

Broad congruence between patients and carers except in relation to presence/absence of psychological symptoms, degree of distress caused to patients by symptoms, and types of main symptoms experienced by patients on admission to hospice.
Congruence for most symptoms; almost perfect agreement for immobility and dyspnoea; substantial agreement for weakness, vomiting/nausea, constipation, and anxiety.

Congruence not high. Relatives generally more critical than patients.

Substantial agreement for immobility; moderate agreement for anxiety and dyspnoea; fair or poor agreement for pain, weakness, vomiting/nausea, constipation, confusion, depression, anorexia, and malaise.

Staff ratings significantly correlated with patient ratings, but staff recorded significantly less severe pain than patients
Broad agreement but staff identified more problems with patient anxiety than patients.

Substantial agreement for immobility; moderate agreement for vomiting/nausea, dyspnoea, confusion; fair agreement for weakness, constipation and depression; poor agreement for pain, anxiety, anorexia, and malaise.

Agreement high for 3 items (practical aid, wasted time, communication of professionals to patient and family); agreement low for pain control, patient and family anxiety, and especially poor for symptom control.

Broad agreement though home carers tended to rate problems worse than staff.

Agreement high for 3 items (practical aid, wasted time, communication of professionals to patient and family); agreement low for pain control, symptom control, patient and family anxiety.

In general, most studies that have examined congruence between patient and home carer accounts conclude that in situations where interviewing patients is impossible or ill advised, then home carers can provide important sources of information about the experience of terminal illness, the extent to which patient symptoms were controlled, and the responses of the health and social services. Home carer accounts are likely to be less useful when assessing patients' quality of life, or examining the severity of anxiety or depression felt by the patient. Of course, not all patients have home carers close enough to be able to report on their symptoms, and even where patients do have spouses or other relatives and friends involved in their care, inpatient admissions during the final months and weeks (hospital, hospice, and nursing home) may reduce the exposure of the home carers to the daily experience of patient care. Nevertheless, patients and home carers both have important stories to tell, even if they do not agree on all points. When it is possible to listen to both, then a fuller picture is painted of the experience of care.

Bereavement care

The aims of palliative care to provide support for the family do not cease with the death of the patient but extend onwards into the time of bereavement (Parkes 1993*a*). Evaluation research can therefore focus on a number of bereavement-related processes and outcomes. First of all, the experiences of bereavement and their impact, as influenced by the care which patients and their families receive during terminal illness, can be examined in a comparative manner, between different sorts of terminal care. Secondly, the effectiveness of bereavement interventions, as provided within the 'palliative care package', may be examined for their effect on outcomes, as well as the efficiency with which they are targeted and delivered.

Dying, death, and bereavement

Research on bereavement and grief has a long tradition in the social and psychological sciences, and there has also been substantial interest in the psychoneuroimmunological pathways involved in the higher morbidity risks that are typically seen in the bereaved.

Descriptive work has focused on the form that grief takes in the weeks, months, and years following bereavement—first of all attempting to classify reactions to bereavement in terms of normal, abnormal, or pathological grief; additionally, exploring the stages through which grief reactions move (normally and abnormally) and also identifying personal and situational factors that appear to influence long-term adjustment. Much of this work has taken place in the UK, the United States, and Australia, and is well reviewed elsewhere (Stroebe and Stroebe 1987; Littlewood 1992; Parkes 1993a; Walter 1994; Hogan *et al.* 1996).

The effects of bereavement on physical health have long been suspected. Surveys carried out in the 1950s and 60s observed excess mortality amongst young widowed people. For example, Rees and Lutkins (1967) found a seven-fold increase in risk between bereaved and control group in their study of mortality amongst close relatives over a six-year period in a semi-rural area in Wales. This increased risk of mortality (from causes other than suicide) amongst the bereaved has been noted in other studies, whilst the precise causal mechanism is unclear. It is hypothesised that depression can cause a reduction in the immune response thus leaving the depressed person more open to infection, but the evidence is not readily forthcoming to support this (Spurrell and Creed 1993). The increased mortality from ischaemic heart disease (IHD) has led to discussion about the role of lipids, although one study failed to show any increase in plasma cholesterol (associated with increased risk of IHD) amongst a group of nine, postmenopausal bereaved widows (Coulter *et al.* 1993).

Despite inconclusive evidence of the neuroimmunological pathways between depression brought about by bereavement and increased mortality, it is generally accepted that bereavement can aggravate or accelerate existing health problems, particularly in the younger age groups of bereaved people. Why younger spouses appear to be greater affected by bereavement could well be a function of the type of death more commonly experienced at younger ages. Situational factors that have been implicated in acute grief reactions include unanticipated and sudden deaths, untimely deaths (that is, deaths of children and young adults), and traumatic deaths possibly due to violence (Parkes 1993b). Personal factors, such as previous psychiatric history and relationship with the deceased and with other family members, have also been found to influence the way in which grief is experienced. The interest in identifying factors associated with increased physical and psychological morbidity is important in the creation of profiles of risk factors, which can be used for screening people either before or after bereavement with the intention of proactively offering bereavement support to those identified as at risk.

In the case of palliative care, most if not all deaths will be anticipated in some way by the relatives as long as the communication has been both honest and open during the course of the terminal illness. According to risk factors that have been identified, some amount of anticipatory grief can have the effect of reducing the intensity of grief after death, and is possibly to be encouraged, although not at the expense of isolating the patient and advancing their 'social death' well before their biological death. Deaths from cancer will generally not be unexpected; some, for example from paediatric cancers and cancers affecting young or middle aged adults, may be untimely. One of the goals of palliative care is to ensure that they are not traumatic. It is often suggested that a death from cancer which is accompanied by uncontrolled symptoms, lack of nursing support, and extreme fatigue in the home carers is a traumatic experience which can lead to intense feeling of guilt, anger, and blame which can complicate the grieving process. From this comes the goal of specialist palliative care to minimize the likelihood of traumatic death through ensuring comfort for the patient and facilitating openness about impending death and ways of coping with it.

An approach to palliative care evaluation could be through the assessment of bereavement outcomes following different forms of terminal care (for example, palliative care compared to conventional care). Assuming that patients who receive specialist palliative care do indeed have a less traumatic terminal illness than patients who do not receive such care, theoretically it should be possible to observe better adjustment to the death, quicker resumption of daily activities, and lower levels of depression. This was basically one of the hypotheses examined by the National Hospice Study in the US, 1978–85, although the study also attempted to differentiate between *home-based* hospice care and *inpatient* hospice care, as well as make the comparison between hospice and conventional care (Sherwood *et al.* 1988). The results only partially supported the hypothesis. The primary care givers of inpatient hospice patients fared better with respect to emotional stress, feelings of burden, and satisfaction with patient care, compared to the home hospice patient care givers, and those of conventional care patients. Further, the care givers of conventional care patients seemed to do better than the carers of home-based hospice patients. The authors suggest that home caring can place a heavier burden on the home carer, which appears to exact a toll in the early months of bereavement (this study examined bereavement outcomes in the first four months of bereavement), but that in the long term, home carers may recover satisfaction at having carried out the home caring task. Other studies have also failed to demonstrate clear evidence of differences in bereavement outcome after different types of care (Seale and Kelly 1997). Even leaving aside the comparison of different types of care; it appears that the assumption that more hospice or palliative care (that is, a bigger dose) might be associated with better home carer adjustment is also problematic. A recent study found no relationship between hospice length of stay and home carer adjustment, although the author states that with the 'omniscience of hind-sight' the hypothesis was probably too simplistic (Speer *et al.* 1995). The research evidence relating to bereavement outcome is clearly not substantial, possibly because relatively short follow-up times (three to six months) do not detect the effect of different care approaches, and possibly also because survey instruments have been insufficiently sensitive.

Models of bereavement support

Whilst it is difficult to study the indirect effects of hospice care on bereavement outcomes, as already discussed, it is also hard to assess the direct effects of bereavement support interventions provided by hospices and specialist palliative care teams. The provision of bereavement support features in the service specifications of palliative care services, as well as being a concern of other health care professionals. Many hospitals increasingly are employing bereavement officers to provide a service for the families of people involved in sudden deaths, perinatal and neonatal deaths (for example, Appleton *et al.* 1993), and accidental deaths, while community-based health care professionals also expect bereavement care to come within their remit. Most specialist palliative care providers have developed bereavement follow-up services, many following the model of the St Christopher's Hospice Bereavement

Support Service which was established in 1970. However, in the UK there is now an extraordinary variety in the type and extent of bereavement support which is provided (Bromberg and Higginson 1996). Without describing these services in detail (see Parkes (1993*a*) for a review of bereavement services), their nature seems to fall into a number of types: provision of information, practical support, emotional support, bereavement counselling and bereavement therapy. These different types of services are provided in individual or group-based ways by health care professionals (nurses, family doctors, community psychiatric nurses, psychiatrists), social workers, professional counsellors, clergy, or volunteers; some of the services are offered as a follow-up, from the settings where the deceased was cared for. Wilkes (1993) carried out a survey of bereavement services offered by hospices and found that just within this sector there was great variety in the form and content of services, as well as in the extent to which hospices kept records of their bereavement service activity and number of clients.

Some evaluations of bereavement support services have focused on process issues, for example, utilization of risk assessment schedules (Payne and Relf 1994), satisfaction with discrete interventions such as memorial services (Foulstone *et al.* 1993), and experiences of bereavement care (Marquis 1996); while others have attempted to compare bereavement outcomes in people who have experienced various kinds of bereavement intervention programs with control groups. Some of these studies have shown a positive effect of bereavement intervention (Raphael 1977; Kay *et al.* 1993; Sadler *et al.* 1992), others have not produced such results (Lieberman and Yalom 1992). There seems to be consensus however in the literature that for 'high risk' individuals, both counselling and psychotherapy can increase the likelihood of relief from pathological or chronic grief (Parkes 1981 and 1986).

Methodologically there are problems with such studies. For example, the choice of outcome indicators may not adequately reflect the changes that are brought about by the intervention, while the process of assessing the control groups is open to interpretation as intervention in itself. The nature of bereavement intervention in the form of focused counselling groups or mutual help groups is influenced by the personalities of the group members, and changes as the personnel changes; such varying group dynamics mean that studies cannot be replicated. Even so, Parkes maintains that 'when

all the problems of evaluating psychotherapies and social interventions are taken into account, the surprising thing is that significant findings emerged at all . . . But there is now good evidence
from several well-conducted studies that those who are especially
vulnerable to bereavement will benefit from a little help given by the
right person at the right time' (Parkes 1986). Wilkes also considers
that 'While acknowledging the difficulties of accurately assessing
the calibre of bereavement services, to offer a service may be of
more help in palliating the sorrows of death than any other activity
in the hospice movement' (Wilkes 1993).

Conclusion

The home carers of terminally ill patients have needs relating to the
period of terminal care, and also afterwards during bereavement.
The aims of specialist palliative care are to identify and meet those
needs in the families of the patients, and this chapter has questioned
how well this happens as reflected in the research literature. As
observers, recipients, and participants in the terminal care process,
home carers have been asked to comment on the satisfaction they
feel with the services provided, from their own point of view and
from the point of view of the patients. Various studies have shown
that home carers express more satisfaction with hospice care than
with conventional care, although gaps in service provision still
exist. Carrying out surveys of bereaved carers can be a useful way of
collecting local information about the adequacy of hospital and
community-based services, but the accuracy of such information is
open to recall bias, and it also raises the question of how grief can
change interpretations of the previous events.

Using bereavement outcomes as indicators of the quality or
effectiveness of specialist palliative care illustrates how involved the
evaluation of such care can become. Incorporating the perspective
of the home carer is important, since social support is a crucial
aspect in the use of professional services and the associated level of
satisfaction. However, this is clearly a complex area, both for the
conceptualization of the issues of importance, and for the choice
of outcome or process indicator. Continuing work in this area,
particularly using prospective research designs, is required.

4

Professional carers

Introduction

An important perspective to take in evaluations of palliative care is that of the professional carer. Palliative care staff are of course the ones who 'do' the palliative care—the engaging, talking, listening, assessing, comforting, and caring. Implicit in all evaluations therefore are questions of how well staff carry out their tasks, how competently they apply their knowledge of symptom control, how empathetically they meet the psychosocial concerns of patients and their home carers, and how efficiently the organizational frameworks within which they work, allow them to fulfil their roles. So, behind the frontage of every palliative care team is a complex organization, with staff performing their caring roles through the interpersonal relationships and hierarchies which structure the service. And because palliative care is not characterized by a limited range of technical procedures, the team itself can be seen as the prime 'intervention'. Teamwork however, is hard work; it actually does matter that compatible staff work together, and it is also important what attitudes and experience staff bring to the specialty of palliative care. Approaches to the evaluation of palliative care services therefore have to be concerned with the evaluation of the clinical and supportive skills of palliative care practitioners and administrators.

The previous two chapters have concentrated on the potential impact of palliative care on patient- and home carer-based indicators (quality of life, symptom control, satisfaction, practical and psychosocial support during terminal illness, and bereavement support afterwards). But how can staff contribute to the evaluation of palliative care? Are they simply commentators on its quality as they perceive it, or is it also necessary to examine the effect of the palliative care profession on the professionals? It could be asked whether palliative care as a specialty exacts an unacceptable toll of stress and burn-out from the staff, and whether specialists in palliative care 'deskill' other medical and nursing professionals. It is suggested in this chapter that these questions are pertinent when wider evaluations of palliative care are considered.

It could be argued that allowing the care of people who are terminally ill to become a medical and nursing specialty is beyond what should be expected of health care professionals. It means that people spend their daily lives constantly in the presence of intense emotion, sadness, and impending death, without the 'dilution' of patients who become cured, or patients with whom it is possible to build up relationships over long periods. What sort of people can cope with this on an extended basis, and does the specialization of terminal care constitute 'over-professionalism' in what should be routine medical and nursing care? There are a myriad of arguments for and against the specialization of palliative care which have been well rehearsed elsewhere (for example, Pugsley and Pardoe 1986). Specialization is a feature of modern clinical care, and the days of the 'good all-rounder' may have passed. However, it is important to ask whether palliative care produces its own casualties; the staff who burn out and are left with personal anxieties and depressions about death, and the concern whether the less specialized care provided by general practitioners and community nurses is less satisfying professionally when certain patients are 'hived' off to specialist carers.

This chapter uses a theoretical model devised by Steinmetz and Gabel (1992) for family physicians as a way of organizing the different issues faced by staff in the provision of palliative care. This model was proposed as a basis for helping physicians to define their role in caring for dying patients, but it is suggested that it can be usefully extended to cover all staff involved in palliative care. The dimensions of the model which will be discussed below are: (1) direct involvement with the patient and family; (2) the needs and development of staff, and (3) co-operation with other professional care givers. Finally, a brief discussion of the way in which staff may be used as patient surrogates complements the section on home carers as patient surrogates in the last chapter.

Direct involvement with the patient and family

There is relatively little work that describes what specialist palliative care staff actually do. There is a tremendous amount of literature on what specialists aim to do in terms of protocols, goals, and standards, and a certain amount on what specialists think they have done, but very little observational and descriptive work has focused on the process of giving care (Seale 1989). Analysis of specialist palliative care records provides a picture of the volume and range of activity, and as it is suggested in the next chapter, this is a source of basic information underpinning much evaluative work. But even from records, there is no clear picture of how staff become involved with patients and their families—just tantalizing glimpses into various patient and family dramas.

Perhaps the greatest volume of specialist palliative care is provided through the work of home care nurses. Many hospice programmes are entirely domiciliary, but considerable numbers of home care nurses also work from inpatient hospice units or hospital teams, while Macmillan nurses (in the UK) can be attached to conventional community nursing teams or specialist palliative care teams. Specialist home care nursing input can be characterized as broadly advisory or participatory (Boyd 1992). All nurses would probably agree that their role is to provide advice on symptom control and psychosocial issues, but differences exist as to the extent of 'hands-on' nursing they feel prepared to carry out.[1] In a study of 12 urban teams in the UK, four carried out hands-on nursing (and wore uniforms), while the other teams felt their role to be limited to specialist advisors (Boyd 1992). Another study of 10 home care teams in the south-west of England found that seven of the teams were primarily for advice only, two would not preclude hands-on nursing, while one team considered hands-on nursing to be part of the service specification (Robbins *et al.* 1994*a*). As Hunt observes, specialist palliative care nurses carry out most of their work through 'talk' (Hunt 1991), and it might be asked, how do they talk, to whom, and what do they talk about?

Clearly, survey methods using structured questionnaires are unlikely to be sufficiently sensitive or flexible to produce an understanding of what could be described as the 'black box' of the caring encounter, and indeed some might ask whether it is possible to

---

[1] In the UK, the Marie Curie Cancer Care Nursing Service is a home nursing service for terminally ill cancer patients. The service provides night and day nursing, by bank nurses, and is accessed through the NHS community nursing services (via the district nurse). The nurses can be thought of as a community resource for specialist palliative care nursing, but do not constitute a multidisciplinary palliative care team.

dissect its 'inner anatomy'. However, the few attempts that have been made to examine the process and content of caring have not only been fascinating, but have also provided important pointers to ways in which specialist staff can learn from a reflective attitude to their 'talking work'. Hunt's study focused on the conversational processes between symptom control team nurses and terminally ill patients and their families during home visits. The five nurses agreed to record their naturally occurring conversations during 272 visits over a three-month period, and using the extended case-study approach within an ethnographic framework, Hunt analysed the conversations. The four main roles identified by Hunt can be compared to the four 'frames' of staff identity discussed by Peräkylä in an analysis of the care, by non-specialist staff, of dying patients in hospital in Finland. Both are presented in Table 4.1.

The similarities between the frames or roles used by staff in dealing with terminal illness in these different settings cannot go unnoticed. Given the fact that dealing with the distress of terminal illness and death on a daily basis is personally demanding, staff

Table 4.1 Four strategies used by staff in the care of terminally ill patients

Hunt (1991)	Peräkylä (1989)
Bureaucratic role *The institutionally structured means through which the nurses presented themselves and did aspects of their work.*	Practical frame *Instrumental work, taking care of necessary daily tasks in the ward.*
Bio-medical role *Focusing on illness, history taking and the assessments and treatment of physical symptoms.*	Medical frame *Knowing the medical situation of the patient and accomplishing the medical intervention.*
Social-therapy role *Dealing with sentiment and 'humanistic' issues, meeting emotional, social, and material needs.*	Psychological frame *Knowing the emotional reactions of the patients, family, and the staff itself, and capable of managing them.*
Friendly, informal role *Efforts to temper the formalities perceived to be inherent in hospitals but inappropriate in home contexts.*	Lay frame *Feeling and experiencing in the face of a fellow man's death.*

require strategies to manage various situations. Hunt describes the way in which nurses move between roles when faced with home carers who themselves felt in need of care. When the wife of a patient told a nurse that she had developed angina and was not so fit herself to look after the patient the nurse responded by focusing on the patient, asking 'Has he lost weight?' Even when the carer replied 'I've lost a bit, yes . . .', the nurse persisted with 'Has your husband as well?'' (Hunt 1991). In a comparable way, Peräkylä describes how the use of the psychological frame is used to manage 'identity disturbances' (difficult behaviour of patients as perceived by staff); 'A patient's deviation from the identity presupposed by the practical frame threatens the daily working order and authority relations on the ward. Through the shift of the frame, the scene is completely reorganized. The patient's deviation is legitimated . . . explained by her anticipatory knowledge of being separated from her family through death' (Peräkylä 1989).

It is commonly stated that in order for medical staff and nurses to feel confident in anything to do with death and dying, or to feel comfortable in dealing with terminal illness, they should have some understanding of death itself; they should also feel confident in opening up and maintaining an effective dialogue (Youll 1989). The work already described, and also work discussed by Walter, seems to suggest that nurses use a variety of communication styles, some of which open the door for the discussion of existential and spiritual issues as well as practical concerns, while other styles keep such a door firmly closed (Walter 1994). Concentrating on strictly practical problems may keep attention from straying towards painful psychological problems, as well as giving nurses a sense of doing something; a point made by James in her discussion of 'carework' in the hospice; 'Physical tasks could be seen to have been finished . . . if the patient looked neat and comfortable, if the sluice was shining clean and if the drug trolley was tidy . . . the work was well done. The sense of control which could be gained from doing physical tasks contrasted with the sense of inadequacy that could so easily be generated when patients or their families were unhappy' (James 1992).

Most the work analysing the communication skills of specialist palliative care staff has focused on nurses, as the largest group of staff. However, extending this research method to observe the conversational styles of other staff working within the specialist team, including volunteers, would allow a more rounded picture of the process of care. For example, home care nurses who fail to elicit and address the existential concerns of patients and families, may be complemented by a social worker or another member of the team who does, and team working styles will arise from negotiated consensus concerning the strengths and weaknesses of individual members. This process was looked at by Reese and Brown (1997) in their observation of the overlap in work of nurses, social workers, and clergy within a hospice programme in Illinois. US. Interestingly, they found that spiritual and psychosocial concerns were the most frequently raised concerns by patients and their families, underlining the important roles that clergy and social workers can play within the palliative care team.

Observing the work of staff who travel to patients' homes is more difficult than observing work within an institution like a hospice, hospital ward, or day centre. Hockey's anthropological treatment of three settings in which death or its aftermath are experienced—a residential home, a hospice, and a bereavement counselling service— provides a series of contrasts of approach to death. Compared with the residential home, the approach of the hospice is observed to foster the idea and experience of transition—moving from this world to beyond. Hockey describes a day-care session provided for people still living at home, and recounts an episode of how the day-care sister organized a slide show of Burn's night and Christmas parties in the hospice, involving past patients and present staff dressed up in costumes. The day-care sister set up the slide show in a ward to include patients who were bedridden—so, all the day-care patients crammed in with four rather ill men. Hockey observes, 'For those who visited the hospice for day-care, the anticipation of a frightening future has been gently advanced in the few slow paces from day-care to ward. The interlude to which they were entertained drew them further forward in a shared retrieval of the familiar names of those who have preceded them.' (Hockey 1990). Hockey attempts to portray an insider's view of the hospice context and in so doing, she sensitizes the reader to the complex interplay of educational, generational, and social backgrounds of patients and staff, and to the role of domestics and auxiliaries, volunteers, and 'hangers-on', against awareness of the regular arrival and departure of the hearse.

Observations of the content of specialist palliative care in hospitals are also few and far between. Studies have focused generally on the hospital care of dying patients, for example Graham and Livesley (1983) examined difficulties in communication with elderly terminally ill patients in a geriatric medical unit and concluded that improvements were needed in the general understanding of patients' needs. Mills *et al.* published an account in 1994 of general hospital care of dying patients in Scotland (the field work was carried out in 1983), with disturbing case-reports of patients being left unattended and with minimal communication with nursing staff. Peräkylä's account of hospital care in Finland focused on the management of dying patients through the use of psychological explanatory frameworks (Peräkylä 1989).

However, Athlin *et al.* conducted a qualitative study in a Swedish geriatric hospital to understand how the primary nursing model could be used for hospice-style care. Relatives and nurses of terminally ill patients were interviewed about what they understood by 'good care', and how far this was delivered through the practice of primary nursing. Relatives were reported to be satisfied with the system but identified the importance to them of being sure that the patients' needs were seen to, especially with regard to pain relief, and of 'knowing' the nurses, which meant having good contact with them and both themselves and the patients being respected as individuals (for example, staff should knock on doors, or leave them alone if they wished it). Staff were in favour of the primary nursing approach (that is, continuity and individualization of nursing care) but regarded it as two-sided; 'it was felt to be stimulating and rewarding, as well as demanding and burdensome' (Athlin *et al.* 1993). Lunt and Neale's (1987) discussion of the care goals set by hospital and hospice staff also comments on the process of hospice care, and indeed how it compares to other forms. This study tested the hypothesis that hospice staff would set more goals covering more areas of patient concern than hospital staff, and that hospice staff would be able to define their goals more quickly. The authors compared two NHS hospices with three general medical and two general surgical wards in a district general hospital, using Kiresuk's Goal Attainment Scaling technique modified for use in terminal care (Kiresuk and Sherman 1968). The results separated the goals set by nurses from those set by doctors, and found that hospital nurses set goals that covered as many issues as hospice nurses, although hospital doctors set fewer goals covering fewer issues than hospice doctors and their nursing colleagues. Since the investigators uncovered variation between the hospice staff with regard to their goal setting, interpretation of the results was complex but they concluded that the study illustrated the need for better communication between doctors and nurses in hospital.

The needs and development of staff

It has frequently been noted that the feelings and fears of dying people can be too painful for professional carers to cope with on a day-to-day basis without considerable support. In a comprehensive review of the literature on stress in hospice and palliative care, Vachon (1995) describes how high levels of workplace stress were identified from the early days of the hospice movement. Interventions designed to address and minimize stress have therefore been a matter of concern for some time, and their success may perhaps now be seen in the lower levels of reported stress amongst palliative care nurses compared to hospital nurses working in areas such as intensive care. Graham *et al.* (1996) found a similar trend amongst UK physicians, with palliative care physicians reporting less stress and more satisfaction with their work than their consultant colleagues from other specialties. This section therefore turns to a consideration of the type of support that is provided for specialist palliative care staff, how effective it is in achieving its aims, and how the professional needs of staff are met through education and training, and through audit.

Support for staff

'Support' like 'care' is a term that is so imprecise that it can mean almost anything, as long as it is positive and helpful. So it is with staff support; it can mean a number of things, but generally something more formal than the sharing of problems which goes on between colleagues in every setting of professional life. Vachon observes that in the early days of the hospice movement, support from colleagues, family, and friends was important, but that more recently, support from colleagues has been found to be more effective (Vachon 1995). Systems of staff support interventions vary from one-to-one models—such as co-counselling, mentoring, or the availability of senior staff to junior staff—to group-based models. Some support systems include the use of psychiatrists, clinical psychologists, social workers, and chaplains; while hospital-based teams may have access to more generic occupational health services. Alexander (1993) describes the range of groups that may be set up, what their objectives are likely to be, and other parameters such as size, whether they should have a leader, and for how long they should run. He makes the point that staff support groups are too important to be allowed to materialize without careful consideration of their aims, methods, or composition, and that enthusiasm for staff support has fuelled 'the naive assumption that collecting staff together once a week is automatically therapeutic. This is simply not true . . . At times a group can degenerate into an empty ritual or, worse, it can become a source of stress in itself' (Alexander 1993).

Studies which have examined the existence and sources of stress amongst palliative care staff have tended to rely on a number of structured, self-rating questionnaires. Alexander's studies of hospice matrons and nurses involved the use of the General Health Questionnaire (Alexander and Ritchie 1990), the Hospital Anxiety and Depression Scale, and the Bortner and Rosenman Scale (Alexander and MacLeod 1992). Another study of nursing stress used the Staff Problem Questionnaire, the Middlesex Hospital Questionnaire, and the Satisfaction with Decision-Making Structures Questionnaire (Harris *et al.* 1990), while Schaerer's (1993) study of doctors' suffering used a questionnaire developed and tested by the researcher, covering items such as feelings and attitude of the doctor, and somatic and psychological consequences. Vachon lists a number of other instruments that have been used to investigate the pressures on staff, including burn-out, coping, death anxiety, and job stress (Vachon 1995).

Fewer studies have sought to assess the effect of staff support interventions using the instruments already described. Harris *et al.* (1990) tested a group of 21 nurses working in a hospital-based palliative care service both before a short in-service educational programme (designed to reduce stress by providing information and the opportunity to share experiences) and again two weeks after the final meeting. Results showed an improvement in perceived support from colleagues and in skills in dealing with the relatives of dying patients, and decreases in anxiety, somatic symptoms, and hysteria— although general stress levels showed no difference, as did job satisfaction. The authors point out the small numbers involved in the study and suggest that a more closely controlled study with a larger sample might provide results of better generalizability. Vachon (1995) also observes that the efficacy of staff support groups has not, on the whole, been evaluated. Most of the work in this area is descriptive rather than comparative, and reports various consensus views of what professionals believe works best for them from their experience, and therefore by extension what is likely also to work for others.

Teamwork

Apart from formal staff support interventions, it is also commonly asserted that working practices within hospices and specialist palliative care teams contribute to increased job satisfaction. Teamwork and team building are concepts lying close to the heart of the hospice philosophy, and the effectiveness of palliative care as a system of care could be assessed through the extent to which teamwork is encouraged and valued. There is not, however, a great deal of research evidence to support the assertion that teamwork is any more effective in specialist palliative care than in other areas of professional life. Indeed, Vachon points out that increasing amounts of workplace stress perceived by palliative care nurses arise through problems with colleagues, implying that lack of agreement over working practices and objectives may be the cause (Vachon 1995).

Engel points out that when people work as a team 'the effect should be organized co-operation—an agreed, planned working together towards a specific, common goal' although he further adds that this 'presupposes that the group of people has agreed on a goal or purpose and on a mutually acceptable plan in which each member is prepared to participate' (Engel 1994). The processes of establishing goals and objectives are fundamental in any setting, and in palliative care, the agreement of objectives between medical and nursing staff may be one area of contention, while agreement with the non-clinical staff (social workers, chaplains, volunteers) as well as complementary therapists may challenge the common goal-setting process further. As far as the author is aware, there has not been substantial research of the composition and functioning of specialist palliative care teams from the point of view of professional collaboration, support, and conflict resolution. While Ajemian describes the features of the interdisciplinary team, and reviews some of the general literature on teamwork and other writings relating to the role of different professionals within the palliative care team (Ajemian 1993*a*), studies of the effectiveness of different team compositions or their management appear to be lacking.

Education and training

Acquiring the skills and expertise involved in palliative care is important for staff to feel confident in their work, and this again is intimately connected to feelings of stress and anxiety. Support for staff by providing access to in-service training, opportunities to learn new skills, and the formal recognition of increasing experience is a fundamental aspect of professional development. In palliative care, just as in other areas of medical, nursing and psychosocial care, it is important to evaluate teaching and learning methods. Being a relatively new specialty, with an evolving and expanding multidisciplinary remit, the challenge of developing innovative and effective educational methods is real (Sheldon and Smith 1996). Many countries have developed a curriculum in palliative medicine for medical students and for higher specialist training (Scott and MacDonald 1993; Coles 1996), and many basic nursing courses now have a specific element on care for the dying, at different levels. In addition, an expanding programme of post-basic specialist training is available (Corner 1993). Training for social workers in palliative care is a developing field, with some countries, such as Denmark, offering focused training in the care of the dying and bereaved; while more generally, postqualifying training is provided by palliative care units or voluntary organizations (Sheldon 1993). In the UK, Cancer Relief Macmillan Fund's sponsoring of social work lectureships in a number of British universities has brought training in psychosocial palliative care up to postgraduate level.

Training in palliative care for clergy is less formal, and tends to occur through visits to hospices, shadowing chaplains, and placements in hospitals. A number of theological colleges in the UK have courses on death, dying, and bereavement, and some hospices have units for pastoral studies to facilitate the exposure of students to multidisciplinary palliative care (Murray 1993). Training for volunteers is also becoming more established as a recognition of their valuable role in palliative care programmes. Ajemian observes that providing training is the first step in demonstrating that the programme is prepared to invest in the volunteer and expects commitment in return (Ajemian 1993*b*). Most volunteer training programmes are run in-house, and, at least in the United States, curricula for volunteer training now exist.

The training of new specialists in palliative care is however a different issue to the provision of ongoing training and support to existing palliative care staff. Many staff move into palliative care without specialist training, and all staff need to be updated in new methods of symptom control, new initiatives in psychosocial interventions, and to refresh skills in communication. The question here therefore is how well does the palliative care profession attend to the needs of its staff? At present there is not a great deal of research literature which comments on this area of palliative care. A recently reported study from New South Wales in Australia examined the professional needs of 108 nurses. Information was collected by postal questionnaire and a follow-up telephone interview; the measures used were a series of questions drawn up by the research team on perceived needs and clinical knowledge. Few of the nurses had postgraduate qualifications in palliative care (10 per cent), although half had qualifications in oncology; and only 25 per cent had worked in palliative care for more than six years. Forty-eight per cent of the sample believed that their training had not prepared them well for the demands of palliative care nursing, with many identifying needs for in-service and postgraduate training. Forty-seven per cent of nurses reported feeling physically exhausted, and 57 per cent reported feeling emotionally exhausted or stressed. Scoring on the clinical knowledge questions was judged to be lower than might have been anticipated, although higher scoring was linked to postgraduate qualifications in oncology and training received outside Australia. The authors expressed concern at their results, and concluded that their study highlighted the need for expanded in-service training, more access to seminars, conferences, and reference material, with particular attention to be paid to the needs of staff working in rural areas (Redman *et al.* 1995).

Against the general acceptance that further training (courses provided in-house and by other institutions, as well as distance-learning packages), regular seminars (in-house and held in other settings), attendance at conferences (national and international), opportunities to undertake research and study leave, and access to research literature (current journals, on-line sources, libraries) are important components of meeting professional needs, there is scant information about how much is available to staff currently working in different settings. A number of publications describing standards in palliative care include sections on specialist education for staff (National Association of Health Authorities and Trusts 1991; Trent Hospice Audit Group 1992), yet very little has been published on whether these intentions have been realized for all staff. In terms of evaluating professional support within palliative care, this apparent gap in the research record warrants attention.

Audit

It could be argued, following on from the last section, that professional needs come within the remit of palliative care audit—the system of 'internal review of technical quality of clinical practice by the professional groups themselves' (Shaw 1993) that has become the flagship of clinical accountability over the past six or seven years. Audit is a requirement of all professional groups operating in the health services today. This section is not about what sort of audit can be carried out in palliative care, nor a discussion about the need for it; there are a number of comprehensive reviews on the subject to which the reader is directed (Higginson 1992, 1993, and 1995). This section aims instead to ask questions about what audit does for the people who do it in terms of fostering teamwork and addressing the concerns and needs of all staff.

Evaluating audit as a system of staff development has not been reported widely, no doubt because audit as an activity is relatively novel and attention is still being directed at what to audit and how, rather than its impact on staff satisfaction and professional development. Indeed, it might be argued that the prime purpose of audit does not lie in this direction. However, it has also been pointed out that for audit to work well, it has to be a team activity, owned by the team, with its objectives and methods agreed by all; so a link between successful audit and effective team work may be hypothesized.

Finlay has pointed out the emotional difficulties for any team starting to appraise its care and the costs in terms of staff time, but concludes from her experience that audit has been a constructive medium through which to identify deficits in care and instigate changes (Finlay 1993). An attempt to assess more formally the impact of audit is reported by Hayes (1993) who evaluated the introduction of audit methods using STAS (the Support Team Assessment Schedule developed by Higginson *et al.*) within a hospice setting. Twelve months after the introduction of the audit system questionnaires were distributed to the doctors and nurses, who were asked to record their reaction to it, what they found most and least useful, and whether they wanted to continue with it. Twenty-one out of twenty-five questionnaires were returned, with 15 respondents stating that they found the audit system useful. Among the beneficial aspects were considered to be the identification of problems and the provision of overviews of patients' progress. The least useful aspects were that audit results fail to show a clear picture of the patient, and the time/workload implications of the exercise. Sixteen considered it was worthwhile continuing, while five wanted to stop because it was too time consuming (Hayes 1993; see also Higginson 1995).

STAS is primarily a method of clinical audit, particularly involving nursing staff, while audit more generally can involve any number of organizational and process aspects across the multi-disciplinary team. Ingleton and Faulkner discussed the implications of multidisciplinary audit with eight senior nurses in the Trent Region (UK), through semi-structured interviews, to canvas opinions of the palliative care standards developed by the Trent Hospice Audit Group. All respondents raised the issue that a planned education programme should accompany the introduction of audit, so that all staff can be well informed of the principles behind the various standards to be audited (Ingleton and Faulkner 1993). A slightly different approach, which has more in common with the procedures adopted in systems of health care accreditation and formal quality assurance, is the organizational audit, carried out by external staff. An example of this kind of audit is that developed in the UK by Cancer Relief Macmillan Fund. Prouse observes that this represents a new direction in palliative care by combining specifically designed standards with a survey of the implementation of those standards by a multiprofessional team of experts in palliative care (Prouse 1994). Audit by a team of experts is clearly a different kind of process to a mutually agreed review agenda set by a small group of practitioners. In this sense, audit will clearly take on different meanings, and come to be viewed as a relevant means of staff support and development in a variety of ways.

Co-operation with other professional care givers

Staff working as specialists in palliative care provide their services alongside those of the mainstream or conventional health services. Most palliative care services indeed rely on referrals from conventional health care providers, and so the question of how satisfied the latter are with the services supplied by the former is of great importance; so too is the question of how co-ordination, communication, and teamwork can best be established between the different care sectors.

How are specialists rated by their non-specialist colleagues?

Most surveys on the views of other health care professionals with regard to specialist palliative care services have focused on the primary care team—general practitioners (GPs) and community nurses. Over the past 30 years there have been a number of surveys asking GPs how they assess their own capacity to care for terminally ill patients (Wilkes 1965; Keane *et al.* 1983; Haines and Booroff 1986; Herd 1990; Wakefield *et al.* 1993; de Maturana *et al.* 1993; Dworkind *et al.* 1994). These surveys have been the basis for various practical and educational initiatives to support GPs in their work, and have also provided some of the *raison d'être* for the establishment of specialist palliative care domiciliary teams (Barritt 1984).

Asking GPs and community nurses how helpful they have found specialist palliative care services is an important way of discovering service gaps and problems. Many of the surveys which have been carried out have reported high levels of satisfaction with specialist services. Table 4.2 presents the results from a selection of studies, highlighting the issues which appear to be problematic. Communication difficulties were identified by many studies, either at the time of referral to the specialist services, or during the period of specialist involvement. In addition, confusion over the respective roles of the specialists and non-specialists has been reported, particularly by community nurses, while frustration with waiting times and delays for inpatient beds in hospices are a continuing theme in some areas. The extent to which specialist services replace mainstream services is more difficult to assess—whether because the former services are viewed as more appropriate for terminally ill cancer patients, or because the latter are considered to be in-adequate. A regional survey carried out by the author (Robbins *et al.* 1994*a*) showed that GP satisfaction with services varied across the nine health districts studied, from 61 per cent of GPs in one health district stating that they always or sometimes had difficulty getting patients into beds for terminal care, to only 22 per cent in another. Disaggregating the effects of inadequate mainstream provision from the satisfaction felt with specialist services because they 'fill in', rather than because of their distinctive contribution to patient care, is not straightforward. However, it is important to know why GPs and community based staff are satisfied with specialist services.

Supporting non-specialists in palliative care

There is a sense within palliative care that specialist services are at the 'disposal' of the mainstream, conventional health care services. Specialists do not necessarily take over the complete care of patients but seek to offer expertise, and provide supplementary and com-plementary care which the mainstream services cannot, or do not, offer. The intention is always to improve the standards of palliative care in all settings, and this involves supplying the appropriate services, offering training and education to non-specialists in the basic principles of palliative care, and also providing general multi-professional, cross-sector support. Perceptions of the services provided have already been discussed, with generally a high level of appreciation expressed by community-based health care pro-fessionals towards specialist services. However, for specialists to be able to work effectively, it is important that awareness of the general principles of palliative care should become more widely understood.

As discussed palliative care is becoming more integrated into medical and nursing curricula, but there is still a need for practising clinicians to be aware of what the specialists can offer, and how their own competencies in palliative care can be improved. Jeffreys' study of the educational needs of general practitioners and community nurses in palliative care found that 87 per cent of respondents (n = 278) felt that their basic or undergraduate training did not prepare them either 'adequately' or 'at all' for caring for dying patients in the community (Jeffreys 1994). Specialist palliative care principles recognize the need to support such professionals but quite how well this is accomplished could also be regarded as a measure

Table 4.2 Views of non-specialist health professionals about specialist palliative care services

Authors	Target group	Response rate	Location	Types of specialist service available	General satisfaction	Issues arising
Copperman (1988)	GPs	226/292 (77%)	London (north), England	Domiciliary hospice team	94% generally happy that the service is available	Improve communication.
Hockey (1991)	GPs, district nurses	220/268 (82%) 68/80 (85%)	Edinburgh, Scotland	Hospice home care team	72% of GPs and 58% of district nurses satisfied with service in present form	Whether to widen referral system to include district nurses. Extension to 24-hour, 7-day per week service—'more of everything seemed to be wanted'.
Sibbald and Simpson (1991)	GPs	192/unknown	London (south), England	Hospice home care team	'Generally satisfied with hospice service'	Younger doctors want more flexible and responsive service (shorter waiting times).
Macdonald and Macdonald (1992)	GPs and consultant	550/341 (62%) (More GPs than consultants)	Ayrshire, Scotland	Reactions to opening of new inpatient hospice	94% of users found hospice helpful; 23% found bed access inadequate	After year of opening 71% of GPs and 60% of consultants had made referrals. Included renal illness as appropriate for hospice care
Boyd (1993)	GPs and district nurses	193/329 (59%) 43/74 (58%)	London (east), England	Hospice home care team	88% of GPs and 86% of district nurses satisfied with service provided by home care team	Multidisciplinary referrals approved but GP should be consulted. Less delay requested in responding to referrals. District nurses in favour of sharing practical nursing care with home care teams. Communication and training improvements needed.

Seamark *et al.* (1993)	GPs and community nurses	127/178 (71%) 58/73 (80%)	East Devon, England	Domiciliary hospice service	'Universal agreement concerning special skills of domiciliary service'	33% of nurses had difficulty knowing who had overall responsibility for patient; 28% of nurses felt their own contribution under-rated. Request for educational courses.
McWhinney and Stewart (1994)	Family physicians	189/245 (77%)	London (Ontario), Canada	Palliative care home support team	'More than two thirds gave the team high ratings'; between 2% and 12% of responses were negative	94% had used the service. Transfer of patient care to team may break continuity of relationships and lead to loss of skills.
Boyd (1995)	GPs	560/705 (79%)	London (south), England	Specialist home care teams	89% rated services as good or excellent	Good liaison with GP highlighted. GP needs to be consulted over hospital to team referrals. More training in non-malignant terminal care.
Robbins *et al.* (1996*a*)	GPs and district nurses	417/578 (72%) 17 interviews with district nurses	South-west England	Specialist palliative care services	87% rated services as satisfactory	Difficulties identified over referral processes and response, lack of beds when needed, poor co-ordination, and conflict over roles.

of the effectiveness of palliative care. Educational programmes for
GPs, district nurses, hospital nurses, nurses working in nursing
homes, social workers, and other therapists have become standard
in many inpatient hospices, and other specialist teams (domiciliary
teams and hospital symptom control teams) also devote considerable
resources to educational outreach. Apart from improving clinical
skills in symptom-control, specialists seek to sustain a change in
attitudes to communication, openness in dealing with death and
dying, and ways of coping with anger and distress in patients and
their families.

There are several ways of providing in-service training to other
professionals, some of which have been evaluated. Nash and Hoy
(1993) described a programme of three-day residential workshops for
GP / district nurse pairs and demonstrated that the workshop format
was highly valued and appeared to increase levels of confidence in
some areas of palliative care (particularly in counselling and communicating bad news for GPs; and in teamwork, symptom control,
and counselling for district nurses). In addition, participants
reported increased levels of support between the two respective
professional groups (GPs and district nurses) based on a better
understanding of the stress factors involved in each others' work.
Macleod *et al.* (1994) provide a short overview of issues in palliative
care education, drawing attention to questions of the best models of
evaluation and the assessment of long-term attitudinal change. They
report the results of a study carried out to evaluate the benefit of
workshops for trainees and principals in general practice, and using
a combination of research approaches (triangulation) they were able
to demonstrate improvements in confidence and coping mechanisms
6–12 months after attendance at the workshops.

Long-term change is an issue that others have examined, and a
recent study reports the results of a three-year follow-up of district
nurses (Jones 1995). Eight district nurses, from different practices,
attended a three-day workshop and then regular follow-up meetings
over the next few years. At the initial workshop they established a
series of objectives which they felt would improve the standards of
terminal care in the community setting, with emphasis being placed
on improving co-operation with GPs and instituting joint reviews.
The small number of nurses meant inevitably that there was some
attrition over the three-year follow-up, and with the lack of a control
group, it is unknown whether the improvements that were reported

were genuinely attributable to the workshop and follow-ups. However, Jones reports that the nurses became more confident in their ability to improve standards of terminal care within the practices in which they worked, at a time of disruption in the management of general practices, and concludes that the district nurses did act as catalysts in improving the process of management of terminal care at home.

A theme emerging from the studies already reported is that participation in workshops fosters an improvement in *confidence* at being able to deal with the challenges of terminal illness, as well as improvement in communication with professional colleagues. Effective communication with patients and families is also important, indeed it underpins good-quality care, but communication skills are not always taught formally as such. Faulkner and O'Neill (1994) point out that most complaints by patients and relatives about medical care relate to communication problems. Communication skills need to encompass communication between staff and patients and their families, interprofessional communication, and also the facilitation of communication between patients and their families. Faulkner and O'Neill (1994) describe the running of five-day workshops for professionals involved in the care of patients with advanced disease (both specialists in palliative care and non-specialists), and report how evaluation has moved from being essentially subjective (postcourse evaluations) to more objective (skills demonstrated at the beginning and end of the course, and six months later) (see also Faulkner 1992).

Staff and patient stories

This chapter has concentrated on assessments of how well specialist palliative care staff are supported, and how their actual work has been perceived. In many ways, these are indirect though important markers of service quality. However, this last section briefly discusses how staff are involved in the more direct assessment of palliative care, and how well staff perspectives reflect those of patients. In a similar vein to the debate concerning the extent to which home carers accurately report patients' concerns, the amount of congruence between staff and patients' views has also been investigated. A number of studies have found that staff generally rate symptoms less severe than patients (Butters *et al.* 1993; Higginson and McCarthy 1993) and anxiety and communication problems more severe (Higginson and McCarthy 1993). These studies have compared the ratings obtained through the Support Team Assessment Schedule (Higginson 1993). In a different approach, Ferrell *et al.* (1993) explored the different meanings of pain to patients and staff through qualitative means. She found that patients understood pain as a multilayered phenomenon, reflecting ultimate and immediate concerns, while nurses were more challenged by the clinical aspects of its management. 'Nurses perceive pain as clinically unnecessary for the patient to experience, yet a clinical challenge to eradicate as efficiently as possible . . .Some patients viewed pain as a challenge with which to live . . . Because the patient equates the intensity of pain with the progression of the disease, he or she can use it as a monitor of the disease.' (Ferrell *et al.* 1993).

Reported perspectives of the severity of symptoms are likely to vary with the methods of measurement. Qualitative approaches to the meaning of symptoms examining, for example, the extent to which they bother a patient, the extent to which staff think they bother a patient, or how much staff feel they would be bothered by the symptoms if they were in the patient's place, will uncover a complex web of objective and subjective evaluations. Measuring symptoms through structured means only allows a limited response, but the resulting picture is that much more clear-cut—though possibly more superficial. Both types of approaches have their limitations and their advantages; using structured instruments may foster a false sense of achieving the goals of palliative care, while qualitative approaches may uncover existential and spiritual concerns which are unconnected to the quality and efficiency of the care being delivered. Knowing what can be obtained through the different methods is clearly important for matching the right method to the chosen research question.

Conclusion

This chapter has uncovered a series of gaps in the research record on professional aspects of palliative care. The literature on palliative care objectives, service specifications, and standards is strong on assertion and rhetoric, but weak on the evidence to back up the claims of what palliative care staff actually do. This may well apply to other clinical specialties too, but in many of these, the relationship between input (for example surgery), output (for example, repairs or excisions), and consequences (for example, reduction of discomfort, return to daily activities) is much clearer. The aims of palliative care are wider than providing expert symptom control when needed, and include 'open communication', caring, support, and so on, which are far more difficult to observe and describe and to attach appropriate outcome measures to.

Qualitative research methods have contributed substantially to the understanding of how staff approach their caring roles and how they adjust to working with people who are dying, and it is hoped that similar future work will provide more insights (Fisher 1996). An appreciation of the tone and character of the caring encounters between both specialist and non-specialist staff with patients and their families is vital for opening the 'black box' of clinical care.

This chapter has tried to draw attention to palliative care staff in a way that emphasizes that they are as much a part of the 'palliative care experience' as the patients and the home carers. Drawing staff into the evaluation of palliative care has to involve more than their commentaries on the adequacy of symptom control; it should also include their professional development needs, and the effectiveness of their own teamworking and collaboration with non-specialist professionals.

5

Service activity and cost data

Introduction

The discussion so far has covered the perspectives of the patients, the family, and the professional staff in the search for process and outcome indicators to be used in the evaluation of palliative care. This chapter now turns to consider the impact of palliative care services at the wider population level. For example, how have palliative care services changed patterns in the place of death of populations and do all sectors of the population get referred to and use hospices? How much do palliative care services cost, and who pays for them? Looking at the effect of palliative care at this level is important for health service planning. Providers need to have an idea of the effect of their services and likely future demand, while health care purchasers need to assess whether services are being provided on an equitable and efficient basis. These are the issues which this chapter is concerned with, involving first, a discussion of the use of vital and routine statistics as commentaries on service activity, and then a review of evidence from surveys which have sought to describe the impact of different kinds of palliative care in various settings. Finally, the question of the costs of different types of palliative care will be addressed, drawing attention to the ways in which such costs have been apportioned between the state, the voluntary sector, and the individual.

Vital and routine statistics

Information about the health of populations and their use of health services can be derived from vital statistics and health service activity data. These are important in the evaluation of health services from an epidemiological perspective, and for informing the strategic planning of health care commissioning agencies. This section focuses on the value of mortality statistics, routine health service statistics, and specialist palliative care service statistics.

Mortality statistics

Deaths have to be certified and registered in most countries of the world, and this allows the compilation of mortality statistics. Death certificates are returned to national clearing houses (for example, the Office of National Statistics (ONS, formerly OPCS) in England and Wales, and the National Center for Health Statistics in the US), where they are coded and statistics compiled. These statistics constitute a vital baseline measurement for the population-based, retrospective assessment of palliative care. Knowing where people died, of what cause, and when, forms the basis of many inquiries. Of course, these statistics are only reliable in as far as the information collected on the registration forms reflects an accurate picture, and at the outset, it is worth drawing attention to some of their possible shortcomings and limitations:

1. *Cause of death*
Deaths have to be certified by a medical practitioner, who enters the main cause of death, and any underlying or contributory causes, on the death certificate. The doctor who certifies death is generally required to have been familiar with the deceased person in the time before death, in order to base the cause of death on sound clinical judgement. In cases of sudden death or where the cause was unclear, certification will be performed by a coroner (or equivalent) after an autopsy. Various authors have pointed out how the value of mortality statistics are jeopardized by inaccuracies in certification, through doctors overdiagnosing certain conditions, such as myocardial infarction, and by variable standards in the autopsy process (Bartley 1985; Bloor *et al.* 1989; Prior 1989; Maudsley and Williams 1996). Not only may the certified causes of death not reflect the true prevalence of such causes in the population, but their transfer into cause of death codes may also further distort the reality, despite the international conventions for cause of death coding (Donaldson and Donaldson 1993). For causes of death involving cancer it is unknown how these processes affect the accuracy of the data. In many cases, a known diagnosis of cancer is less likely to leave room for inaccuracy in cause of death although there may be a

chance of inaccuracy relating to the primary site of the tumour. Support for these observations come from the fact that neoplasms are amongst the least likely of diseases to be certified by a coroner (implying greater confidence in the cause of death), and also many of the medical enquiries sent out by the ONS, for example, requests for more information from certifying doctors (3 per cent of all deaths), have been related to the redefinition of the sites involved in deaths ascribed to cancer (Ashley and Devis 1992). Overall, it can be assumed that causes of death relating to cancer may be less prone to inaccuracies than other causes of death, such as those due to circulatory problems.

2. *Actual place of death*

Cartwright and Seale (1990) drew attention to possible inaccuracies in death certificate data over place of death, particularly when deaths occurred in public places or in residential homes. People suffering sudden fatal conditions or accidents in public, who are taken by ambulance to hospital, may be certified as having died in hospital although they were actually dead on arrival. Likewise, the coding of deaths occurring in residential homes, and even nursing homes, have been attributed to the 'death-at-home' category, especially if the care home is stated as the usual place of residence. While it is factually correct that a setting which is lived in for over six months becomes the usual place of residence, deaths occurring in a long-stay institution are different, in terms of service planning, to deaths occurring in the domestic home. It is also observed that since the addresses of residential and nursing homes resemble private addresses, institutional deaths can be attributed wrongly to the home category by death certificate coders, even when the institution was not the usual place of residence (Cartwright and Seale 1990).

3. *Place of death codes*

In the UK, the place of death is written on the death certificate but when it is coded, a separate code is not provided for deaths in hospices. Because hospices are registered as nursing homes under the 1984 Registered Homes Act, deaths occurring in these places are submerged within the number of deaths occurring in nursing homes.

4. *Linkage with other datasets*

Also in the UK, because the National Health Service number has never been widely used, there is no easy way to link mortality data with, for example, hospice records or other health service records.

5. *Identifying people with palliative care needs*

The broad remit of palliative care, responding as it does to symp-tomatology and psychosocial needs, means that indications for palliative care are not clear-cut. Traditionally, specialist palliative care has been offered to people who are terminally ill with cancer. However, not all these people require such care, and increas-ingly, specialist palliative care services are made available to other patients who are terminally ill with non-malignant conditions. Like cancer, some of these non-malignant conditions (for example, motor neurone disease) have a fairly predictable course which in-volves a period of terminal illness, requiring attention to symptom management, while other conditions take a far less expectable route. Identifying all the cases by death of certain conditions (for example, people who died of stroke)—through the International Classification of Diseases (ICD) codes, which are used for categorizing the cause of death in mortality data[1]—will vastly overestimate the need for the kind of care offered by specialist palliative care services. For these reasons, using mortality statistics which relate only to cases of death involving cancer is unsatisfactory because it leads to overestimating of the need for palliative *cancer* care, and underestimating the need for palliative *non-cancer* care—although it is a pragmatic approach and widely used.

6. *Local surveys of death certificates*

Regional- or district-based researchers may compile their own statistics directly from death certificates (with appropriately gained access). This can have the benefit of being able to note hospice deaths where they occur, as well as collecting additional information relating to the cause of death if needed. There are disadvantages to this method however, apart from the time and expense of processing the certificates. A study of patterns of death amongst the residents of a health district (generally the population of most interest in terms of health care planning and purchasing) will also need to ensure that information is collected on those who have died in other health districts (transferable or 'out-of-district' deaths). Details of these deaths are not always easily available, and depending on the location

---

[1] The Health Care Financing Administration in the US announced in Autumn 1996 the inclusion of a new diagnosis code for palliative care in the International Classification of Diseases, 9th Revision, Clinical Modifications. This may facilitate the development of a palliative care Diagnosis Related Group (DRG) (Cassel and Vladeck 1996).

of the district (in particular, if it is a metropolitan borough), information could be lost on up to one fifth of deaths (Fleissig and Grant 1984). This could be particularly true of cancer patients being treated at tertiary referral centres in other districts.

This is not an exhaustive list of the problems with mortality statistics, but the points raised draw attention to the caution with which routinely compiled statistics need to be approached. Despite their shortcomings, they can be used for tracking patterns in place of death from cancer and, when combined with other information, may also comment on the likely impact of the specialist palliative care services. To illustrate this the next section describes how mortality statistics may be used to assess the impact of inpatient hospice provision and specialist home care nursing services.

Deaths at home

One of the objectives of palliative care is to enable people to die in as homely an environment as possible; if a home death is not possible, then death in a hospice or in hospital with appropriate specialist input, is also considered an appropriate option. A question to be asked therefore is whether specialist palliative care services have had an effect on the number of people with cancer dying at home?

Mortality statistics currently reveal that around 25 per cent of people dying of cancer die at home, compared to 21 per cent for non-cancer causes of death (OPCS 1992). Patterns in the place of death are sensitive however to regional, district, local, urban, and rural influences. For example, the proportion of people dying of cancer at home in nine districts across the south-west of England were found to range between 20 and 33 per cent; while at electoral ward level, enormous geographical variation was observed for deaths in 1993, with proportions ranging between 50 and 13 per cent (Robbins *et al.* 1994*a* and *b*).

Over the 1980s, inpatient hospice units and home care nursing teams became established in many districts and it might be hypothesized that one of their main effects should have been on the proportion of people dying at home and also in hospital (with hospice deaths replacing inappropriate hospital deaths, and home deaths being supported by the home care nursing services). Proportions of home deaths generally have been declining over recent years—partly explained by the ageing demographic profile and the increase in people living alone (Seale 1991). However, data from 10 health districts in the south-west of England examined by the author, revealed an interesting picture of interaction between inpatient hospice provision and place of death. Mortality statistics were obtained for the years 1981–91 and trends in the place of death of people who died of cancer were examined. The patterns in three of the districts are presented in Fig. 5.1. These graphs show the trends in place of death of district residents who died of cancer over 11 years. Since these figures were derived from routine mortality statistics, inpatient hospice deaths could not be separated from deaths that occurred in nursing homes. Throughout the 1980s increasing numbers of deaths have occurred in nursing homes, although this trend was more marked for people dying of non-cancer causes. However, this is background information that should be kept in mind when assessing the increase in hospice deaths.

Although residents in district A (see Fig. 5.1(a)) had access to hospice services in an adjoining district, during the 1980s there were no actual inpatient hospice services located within the district. Trends in place of death were relatively constant with a comparatively high rate of home death (around 31 per cent) and hospital death (around 54 per cent). The effect of opening an inpatient hospice with 14 beds in district B (see Fig. 5.1(b)) in 1987 is quite marked: both home deaths and hospital deaths declined—home deaths dropped from 30 per cent in 1986 to 24 per cent in 1988, while hospital deaths dropped from 61 per cent in 1986 to 52 per cent in 1988. In district C (see Fig. 5.1(c)), the opening of hospice beds in 1982 may have accounted for a drop in home deaths from 37 per cent in 1981 to 28 per cent by 1983; and after the expansion of the hospice service in 1988, home deaths declined further to 24 per cent by 1990—a change over nine years of 13 per cent. Although unable to comment on the *appropriateness* of these changes, and the extent to which patient and family preferences were met, it is clear that changes did take place in districts with inpatient hospice services and that these changes were able to be monitored by mortality statistics.

Johnson and Oliver (1991) also noted how the introduction of specialist palliative care services in north Kent influenced the place of death of cancer patients. The introduction of a domiciliary symptom control team was followed by an immediate rise in home deaths, which declined after three years (by 1980); while the opening of the

Service activity and cost data

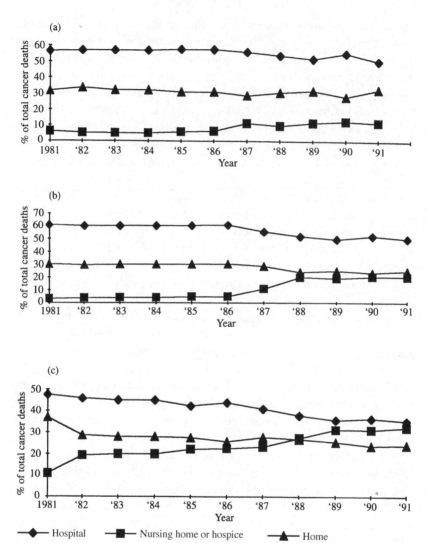

Fig. 5.1 Patterns of place of death of people who died of cancer in three districts: (a) district A—no inpatient hospice or home care nursing service actually located within district; (b) district B—hospice home care service started in 1982 and 14 inpatient hospice beds opened in 1987; (c) district C—seven inpatient hospice beds opened in 1982, increased to 20 beds in 1988.

inpatient hospice in 1984 was followed by a fall in both hospital and home deaths. The downward trend in home deaths reversed after the third year. Thorne *et al.* (1994) showed how place of death is influenced by other service factors such as the availability of general practitioner community hospital beds. Many of the more rural health districts in the UK have retained the small cottage or community hospitals which are mainly used for non-acute care (convalescence, care of the elderly, psychogeriatrics, and also terminal care). Medical care is generally provided by the patients' own GPs. Thorne *et al.* identified all cancer deaths within Exeter Health District (which at that time did not have an inpatient hospice) by examining all the death certificate returns over a one-year period. They noted that access to community hospital beds was associated with a significant decrease in home deaths (29 per cent amongst those whose GP had access to community hospital beds, compared to 41 per cent amongst cancer patients who had no access). They also noted that patients were less likely to die in an acute care hospital if their GPs had access to community hospital beds.

A greater potential for describing patterns in place of death from mortality statistics occurs when they are linked to hospice activity data. For example, place of death comparisons *can* be made between people referred to hospice services and those not referred. Taking an example again from a district in south-west England, a significant difference in likelihood of dying at home was observed for people who were referred to the hospice home care nursing service. In 1993, out of the 1257 people who died of cancer, 464 were referred to the hospice home care nursing service. Thirty-four per cent of these people died at home compared to 22 per cent of those who were not referred (Robbins *et al.* 1996*b*). This does not necessarily prove, however, that the home care service was the sole causal factor in these people dying at home; an unknown proportion would have died at home without referral to the home care service. Younger people tend to die at home because they are more likely to have home support, and it is usually the younger patients with cancer who are referred to the hospice services. This confounding of prior probability to die at home with referral to hospice services has been a feature of many evaluations of hospice care, including the National Hospice Study (Mor 1988).

These examples illustrate how mortality statistics, in combination with other data sources, can be used in the evaluation of hospice services. They comment on past patterns of activity, but cannot pass judgement on the appropriateness of those patterns without more in-depth study (Seamark *et al*. 1995). In an interesting commentary on people who died 'alone' (either because they were unmarried, had no family, lived alone or died suddenly), Seale (1995) suggests that for some people, hospitals may be preferred as places to be when death approaches, rather than facing the prospect of a lonely death at home. However, mortality statistics can at least provide an indication of the volume of terminal care that is likely to be delivered in the different settings. As well, in the controlled evaluation of a home care intervention, they may constitute a relatively 'hard' measure of a targeted palliative care effect, particularly if patient choice in relation to preferred place of death is being monitored.

Routine health service activity data

The potential interest to be gained from analysing routinely collected data is not always completely realized. Within the NHS, there is considerable variation in the quality, volume, and breadth of routine data (Kind 1988). However, with the increasing computerization of hospital index and administration systems, and of general practice, community nursing, and pharmacy records, there is the potential for record linkage across a variety of health service datasets. This could raise the possibility of tracking patients' utilization of health services, and tying this in to evaluations of the best models of care. There is a wide literature now on variation in the use and supply of health services in North America and Europe, and one of the questions facing health services researchers is what such variation actually means in terms of patient outcomes and associated costs.

The usefulness of routine health service activity data in commenting on the utilization of palliative care services varies according to local systems and the extent to which (a) palliative care interventions are recorded and (b) palliative medicine is recognized as a clinical specialty within the health care provider unit. Researchers are recommended to explore local routine health service activity data sources in some detail, as many clinicians have adopted 'stand-alone' audit systems as well as systems that are common to a district or region. The value of the minimum contract dataset—which holds the minimum number of hospital activity data items in the UK—is likely to lie in the quantification of inpatient admissions rather than description of their contents. The ONS/OPCS operation codes that indicate the type of intervention carried out during inpatient admissions can rarely be linked to an episode of palliative care, and even the ICD codes give little indication of the numbers of patients requiring palliative care. As already noted, these codes are based on disease categories, not on symptomatology (or psychosocial problems). Routine health service activity data are also likely to be more comprehensive for inpatient admissions than outpatient care. Much palliative care is delivered in the outpatient setting (for example, lymphoedema clinics, pain clinics) and for routine NHS data at least, diagnosis and procedure codes have only recently become available in outpatient data files (although this varies from unit to unit).

Data relating to the activity of specialist palliative care providers can also be regarded as routine, and this source of information is important both for research and audit purposes. In the UK, recent progress has been made nationally towards the creation of minimum datasets for hospices and specialist palliative care teams (NCHSPCS 1995c). This has drawn attention to the inadequacies in some systems to produce the information required by health care purchasers for contract setting and monitoring. Understandably, though regrettably from the point of view of researchers, many hospices and palliative care teams have followed their health service counterparts in producing data relating only to episodes of care, without the completeness of data capture to allow patient-based care to be described. Circumnavigating this deficiency generally entails manual data abstraction from patients' notes which is immensely time consuming—partly because of the nature of the task, but also because medical and nursing records are not always where they should be.

Health service and hospice data become much more interesting, particularly to health care purchasers and planners, when they can be linked to each other, and the care that patients receive can be tracked across different settings. Doing this helps to understand the extent to which specialist palliative care services interdigitate with mainstream services. Specialist palliative care providers vary in their information systems and the extent to which these can link into secondary and primary care databases. Those working within the NHS (for example, 18 per cent of overall hospice provision is through 595 hospice beds in 56 NHS hospice units (Hospice Information Service 1997)) will have information and computing support from their trust unit, and all their records may well be contained within the central patient administration system. Some independent hospices outside the NHS have moved towards developing on-line links with their local trust units—but many teams stand very much alone.

In the absence of routine data pooling, record linkage techniques may be applied which match records from different datasets. In some areas of the UK (for example, in Scotland) this is done routinely; in other areas, it is not. This method has been used by the author to link mortality data with hospice and hospital records, so that for a cohort of health district residents who died of cancer in 1993, information is available on all the inpatient hospital and hospice input (inpatient, home care, and day care) that these people received in the year before their death. Linkage was achieved in this instance using software developed by the Oxford Record Linkage Project, which has, over the past 20 years, been developing the technique of matching records from different datasets (Gill *et al.* 1993). Matching is carried out on a number of person identifiers (such as date of birth, post code, name (if available) and sex) according to rules of probability. Accuracy of matching can achieve a very high level (over 96 per cent) which compares well with the 'fuzzy' matching available within the more common statistical software packages. Using a numerical identifier on all health and social records would obviate the need for dedicated record linkage exercises, and with new NHS numbers being introduced in the UK, record linkage may be considerably simpler in years to come.

Tracking health service utilization by patients can provide insights into which patients are referred to specialist palliative care services, and the characteristics of those who are not. Specialist palliative care providers rarely know whether they are meeting all the needs for their services within an area. It is now estimated that specialist palliative care services are involved in around 50 per cent of all cancer deaths (Johnson and Oliver 1991; Bennett and Corcoran 1994). Many people who die of cancer obviously do not receive the input of specialists, and it is unknown whether this is because their palliative care needs are adequately met by the primary health care team and hospital services, or whether it is because they do not want specialist palliative care input, or whether they fail to be referred, when they might have benefited from and appreciated extra support. For example, investigating the extent to which GPs refer patients to hospice services can help to assess whether there are likely to be 'pockets' of cancer patients in some areas who stand a very low chance of being referred. This can be done in a limited way from hospice records; comparing the number of GPs represented amongst the cohort of patients referred to the service over a specified period against the known number of GPs within the catchment area. However, it is also interesting to know how many patients are not referred by GPs as well, in order to explore the pattern of referral activity.

Figure 5.2 shows the results of work carried out by Robbins, *et al.* (1996*b*) on linking records from different datasets to examine patterns of hospice utilization against the general characteristics of deaths involving cancer. The data are based on 1207 health district residents who died of cancer in 1993 (87 per cent of the total number of deaths involving cancer) and who had at least one inpatient hospital admission during the year before their death. The health district, located in south-west England, has a population of around 420 000, and has one independent hospice offering 16 inpatient beds, a day care service, hospital liaison, and a home care nursing service. In 1993 there were 290 GPs working in an area slightly larger than the health district area (the family health services authority area was not coterminous with the district health authority area at that time). Of these, 247 were stated to be the GP of 1200 patients who

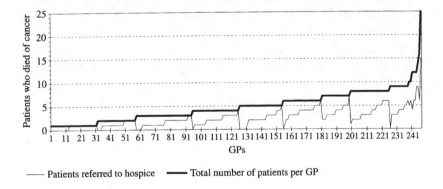

Fig. 5.2 Ranked GPs according to number of cancer patients cared for, and number referred to hospice services.

died of cancer in 1993, during the last hospital admission before their death (seven patients were not registered with any GP). The heavier upper line on the graph in Fig. 5.2 shows the variable number of cancer patients looked after by individual GPs (ranked according to numbers of cancer patients under their care). Just over 30 GPs had only one patient who died of cancer during the year, while one GP (practising in a coastal retirement area) had 25 patients, and 48 GPs had eight or more patients. The median number of patients per GP was four. The lighter line on the graph shows the number of patients 'belonging' to each GP who were referred to the hospice services (and as, Fig. 2.1 on page 47 shows, this could mean a range of services over varying lengths of time). From Fig. 5.1 it can be seen that *all* the patients of 34 GPs, who subsequently died of cancer, were referred to the hospice (those GPs where the lighter lower line meets the upper line), while there were 27 GPs who had *none* of their patients referred (those GPs where the lighter lower line meets the × axis). However, many of these GPs had only one eligible patient (19 whose single patient was referred, and 12 whose single patient was not referred). Overall, 603 patients were referred to the hospice services, which represents about 50 per cent of patients who died of cancer.

Data presented like this give little indication of the appropriateness of referrals or non-referrals, nor who actually did the referring of patients (referrals should not go ahead without the consent and knowledge of the GP, but the GP him or herself might not actually *initiate* the referral), but they do demonstrate that most GPs within this particular health district are actually using the hospice services— and some are obviously using the services more than others. It could be an indication of unequal access to the hospice services or widespread antipathy or dissatisfaction of local GPs if, for example, the data were to show a much higher proportion of GPs not allowing the referral of any of their patients.

Surveys of service structure and function

Linking health records as described in the previous section has obvious potential for the evaluation of specialist services. However, a substantial amount of evaluative information can also be obtained about the structure and function of services by carrying out service-specific surveys. Three main types of service activity associated with specialist palliative care will be discussed: inpatient hospices, home care services, and hospital-based services.

Hospice care

The rapid expansion of the hospice sector after 1970 saw a short period when comparatively little was known about how many palliative care teams were springing up, and what their respective roles were. In 1981, Lunt and Hillier published one of the first surveys of hospice services in Britain, and since then a substantial amount of work has been published describing the work of different teams, estimates of their costs, and so on. Currently, much of the information about specialist palliative care services is collated and disseminated on a national basis in the UK by the Hospice Information Service. This service was established in 1977 at St Christopher's Hospice in London, and is now partly funded by the Cancer Relief Macmillan Fund. The Information Service publishes an annual directory of hospice and palliative care services in the UK and Ireland, as well as a directory of palliative care services worldwide and a range of fact sheets (Hospice Information Service 1997). The summary statistics produced by the Information Service allow comparisons between health districts and regions in terms of the number of specialist palliative care beds per head of population, and the range of palliative care services.

Lunt and Hillier's survey drew attention to the regional inequalities in inpatient hospice provision in 1980—ranging from 10.9 beds per million population in the Trent region to 48.5 beds per million in south-west Thames; and no home care nurses in Mersey and Wales, while Wessex had 5.1 nurses per million (Lunt and Hillier 1981). They suggested that a figure of 45–50 inpatient hospice beds per million population might constitute an adequate level. By 1990, the survey of Smith *et al.* (1992) from the Hospice Information Service showed that although regional inequalities persisted (on the mainland of Britain the provision ranged from 67 beds per million in Yorkshire region to 30 beds per million in Wales; whilst in Northern Ireland, the Southern Board had only 24 beds per million) a median of 45 beds per million had been achieved across much of the country.

In addition to the issue of regional variation in the provision of services, there has been considerable interest in describing the services offered by hospices. A survey carried out in the late 1980s of 98 inpatient hospices tried to describe the work of a 'typical' hospice (Johnson *et al.* 1990). The survey revealed that most hospices (70 per cent) provided a home care service, although many of these teams did not supply 24-hour or weekend cover. The amount of senior medical cover varied: full-time consultants were employed in 76 per cent of the 17 NHS hospices; whilst in independent hospices, 43 per cent had full-time and 42 per cent had part-time consultant staff, and 15 per cent had medical cover provided by part-time general practitioner clinical assistants or local GPs. The authors observed that 'it is difficult to imagine that units that vary so widely in their throughput (1.7–31.8 deaths and discharges per bed per year) and in their discharge rates (1–76 per cent) have much in common other than their title of hospice' (Johnson *et al.* 1990).

The Hospice Information Service has now published the results of five surveys, covering the years from the early 1990s onwards (Eve *et al.* 1997). Their results also show wide variation between the service activity of different hospices, home care teams, day care services, and hospital support services. Hospices vary in terms of numbers of beds, patient lengths of stay, ratios of qualified to unqualified staff, and in terms of the composition of the multidisciplinary teams. Another study also observed that 'Different funding levels, different staffing levels, different catchment populations and different operational policies make it impossible to make direct comparisons between independent hospice units, even when allowance is made for the number of beds' (Kirkham and Davis 1992). The authors of this study drew attention to the difficulty of evaluating hospice activity according to measures of throughput or bed occupancy, since in palliative care it cannot be assumed that simple measures of patient numbers reflect either efficiency or effectiveness. Their point underlines the importance of interpreting the clinical relevance of statistically significant findings. Since palliative care is dependent on the giving of time, increasing patient numbers may be seen as efficient in one sense, but clinically inefficient in another (Kirkham and Davis 1992).

Domiciliary care

The question of who actually gets referred to specialist palliative care services is also linked to the question of who gets referred to what kind of hospice service (if there is a choice). A retrospective review of all patients cared for by St Joseph's Hospice in London during the first six months of 1988 showed that patients referred to the home care service were younger and more likely to be married, and that home care patients were likely to have longer prognoses and to die at home (Dunphy 1990). Two studies from Australia of the characteristics of patients referred to different kinds of palliative care services both showed that the patients referred to inpatient services were older, had more nursing needs, and were less likely to have someone to care for them (Komesaroff *et al*. 1989; Bradshaw 1993). The study by Komesaroff *et al*. also showed that socio-economic differences could be detected—hospice inpatients were more likely to be of the non-professional class; while home care patients were more likely to have had private insurance and have been employed in a professional or non-manual occupation. The studies draw attention to the possibility that different types of palliative care service may be more appropriate for some patient groups than others and to the question of equal access to such care for all groups. A number of studies in the US and UK have looked at the access of patients from minority groups to palliative care (Gordon 1996; Hill and Penso 1995) with the conclusion that they are under-represented.

The general surveys of hospice services referred to have demonstrated the variety in form of domiciliary provision: home care nursing teams may be attached to an inpatient hospice unit or be free-standing; they may offer 24-hour, seven-day-a-week care, or just weekday care; they may provide 'hands-on' nursing care as well as advisory support; some teams may have medical backup; and some teams now make available respite care at home or hospice at home (a comprehensive 24-hour service, including practical nursing and night sitting, provided by a multiprofessional team with access to consultant advice) (Hospice Information Service 1995). The variability between teams raises questions about the value of comparing different services, and what can be gained from such an exercise. If forms of service provision are indeed so heterogeneous, results from one assessment may not be generalizable to other services. Cross-service comparison may be contrasted to the approach of Doyle (1991) who reported on an evaluation of a single home care service over its first 10 years of operation.

Hospital care

The first hospital support team in the UK was established in St Thomas' Hospital in London in 1976 (Bates *et al.* 1981), although this was based on a model already developed in North America (Mount 1976). Since then, many teams have developed in hospitals and, as well, many nurses now work as palliative care support nurses or hospice liaison nurses within hospitals (the current total stands at 176 hospital support nurses and 139 hospital support teams in the UK and Ireland) (Hospice Information Service 1997). Eve and Smith's survey relating to services in 1991 examined the composition of hospital support services and discovered that the results could not be analysed quantitatively because of the varying nature of the work of the different services (Eve and Smith 1994). It was found that some teams took referrals of patients from hospital and followed them up at home, working more like a domiciliary service, while others worked simply within the hospital, visiting patients on wards and in clinics. Some teams, particularly those attached to oncology departments, started patient contact at the time of diagnosis.

A small number of evaluations of hospital-based palliative care teams have been reported to date, looking at several issues including the extent to which teams influence general levels of palliative care within hospitals, and also the work of surrounding community-based palliative care services (Ellershaw 1995; McQuillan *et al.* 1996). One study that has assessed the latter issue is that reported by Bennett and Corcoran (1994). They examined the impact of the setting up of a hospital palliative care team on the community-based palliative care services in Leeds over a four-year period, and noted an increasing referral to death interval. This appeared to have been caused by the earlier referral of patients to the community services by the hospital palliative care team. The implications of this for the workload of the community-based services are considerable, and the authors predict that the numbers of patients referred are likely to rise, and the length of input will increase as well.

Measurement of costs

Evaluating specialist palliative care services in terms of their cost effectiveness and efficiency has become a matter of some interest in recent years. Palliative care services have developed most quickly in Europe, North America, and Australasia over the past 30 years—although often in a relatively unco-ordinated manner. Due to their popular appeal, hospice services have been able to expand, in a time of general financial retrenchment, with funding from charitable foundations, considerable amounts of public fund-raising, and substantial amounts of volunteer help. Although many palliative care services are now provided within mainstream, national health services, much of the innovative clinical and psychosocial work in terminal care was developed, and continues to be developed, in independent settings. This is part of the reason for the marked variation in range and type of palliative care provision that has arisen between localities and regions, as already noted. However, the increasing integration of the voluntary hospice / palliative care sector into mainstream care, and the more widespread adoption of the palliative care approach, raises questions about the overall levels of funding for palliative care, and what model of palliative care (or combination of models) offers the best quality care for dying patients and their relatives, and is also financially sustainable in the future. Underlying these policy issues is the question of how the costs of specialist palliative care services have been assessed, and what conclusion can be drawn about their cost effectiveness. This section therefore reviews some of the evidence relating to the cost assessment of palliative care, while the next chapter considers the question of best models of care.

Considerably more interest in assessing the costs of palliative care has been evident in the US rather than the UK, due, no doubt, to the financing of the American health care system which is insurance based rather than centrally funded from public taxation. When insurance companies took on the funding of palliative care services there was more attention to the prediction and containment of costs, as well as value for money. During the late 1970s and early 80s, hospice care was regarded as a way of reducing those costs of terminal illness associated with inappropriate high technology, and aggressive hospital care. It was believed that the emphasis on less aggressive, interventionist, acute hospital care would bring cost savings. Partly on this assumption Medicare (insurance coverage for those over 65) extended its cover, in 1983, to include care provided by hospice programmes. Evaluations since the early 1980s have failed to demonstrate persistent cost savings of specialist palliative care over conventional care, apart from savings associated with home hospice programmes. Even here, the results have been equivocal with evidence seeming to show that recipients of home hospice services were low utilizers of the health services anyway (Kidder 1988).

Most of the cost comparisons of hospice care and conventional care have been carried out in the US (for example, Kane *et al.* 1984; Brooks and Smyth-Staruch 1984; Kidder 1988) or in Australia (Gray *et al.* 1987; Dunt *et al.* 1989). In the UK, Hill and Oliver published two reviews of the costs associated with hospice care; their findings related to 20 inpatient hospices in the first survey (1984), and 40 hospices in the second (1989). They focused on interhospice cost differences, rather than differences between hospice and conventional care. Certain cost efficiencies were found with the cost per bed per week being higher in units with lower numbers of beds, while costs rose with units having over 30 beds. Overall, the authors stated that they were unable to comment on whether hospice care was cheaper than hospital care, or whether NHS hospice care was cheaper than independent hospice care due to incompatible and unavailable data (Hill and Oliver 1984 and 1989). A research team in Scotland has also attempted to calculate the cost of hospice care using two methods. First, they carried out a survey of 11 hospices, and examined volunteer input, admissions, services, staffing details, and so on, but were unable to come to sound conclusions because of differences in accounting practices between the hospices (King *et al.* 1993). The next approach was to carry out an in-depth study of two hospices (a NHS one and an independent one), calculating costs on an episodic basis by measuring the expenditure involved in caring for individual patients. The study took into account direct and indirect costs, and fixed overheads. Overall costs between the two hospices were not found to be substantially different, however medical overheads were larger in the NHS hospice, whereas administrative costs per patient were four times higher in the independent hospice. More time was spent by staff in the independent hospice in direct patient care, although there was great variability in per capita costs within and between units (Tierney *et al.* 1994). Other studies comparing the costs of different palliative care services include that of Ventafridda *et al.* (1989), who demonstrated the cost savings of home care over hospital care (with input from a palliative care team) in Italy, and also that of Raftery *et al.* (1996) referred to earlier (see p. 50). This latter study demonstrated that a nurse co-ordination service was cost-effective and that this had implications for palliative care services, since co-ordination is a task sometimes taken on by palliative care teams.

In general, economic evaluations of palliative care are hindered by (a) the difficulty in calculating the direct medical and non-medical costs, as well as the indirect costs—especially since many palliative care services rely on considerable and variable amounts of volunteer input; and (b) the lack of evidence of the effectiveness of specialist services (Normand 1996). Because of this, both costs and benefits (or consequences) are difficult to calculate. In the absence of comparative quality of life data or preference / utility data, cost-effectiveness and cost-utility evaluations are also hampered. The assumption that in comparison with conventional care, palliative care should cost less in order to be seen as effective is probably ill-founded. Generally, the greatest cost component during terminal illness is bed occupancy and nursing time. The practice of palliative care generally involves increased levels of nursing and medical and psychosocial assessment, and inpatient hospice care is characterized by high staff to patient ratios. Thus, those aspects of care which account for the major costs of terminal illness are those aspects which palliative care services seek to maximize. In the future, it is important to focus attention on those ways of valuing palliative care which emphasize quality of life rather than quantity.

Conclusion

This chapter has focused on population-based indicators such as place of death and patterns of service utilization, and has suggested that with various caveats, such indicators are sensitive to the impact of palliative care services. Patterns of health service utilization are of course bound up with the service costs, and the chapter finished with a brief overview of the main themes in the literature on palliative care costs. Inpatient hospice provision appears to have the greatest impact on place of death, and in some areas in the UK, as many deaths from cancer occur in hospices as they do at home. The costs of inpatient hospice care are difficult to assess, and may be interpreted in different ways. Because hospices receive a substantial amount of their revenue (on average about 50 per cent) from charitable sources (charitable foundations, fund-raising, donations, and legacies), as well as accruing cost savings through the use of volunteer labour, they provide a subsidized service to health district residents in terms of the costs borne by the statutory sector. However, when undertaking an overall cost assessment of palliative care services, it is important to look at total costs, because even charitable funding has an opportunity cost.

6

Tackling the evaluation of palliative care

Introduction

The preceding chapters have not only attempted to *describe* the evidence base for palliative care, but also to *identify* gaps in the current research record. A range of evaluation strategies have been discussed, and important perspectives have been highlighted. This final chapter has the following aims: first, to draw some lessons about the strengths and weaknesses of evaluation research, and to suggest ways in which the effectiveness of evaluation studies can be enhanced; and second, to examine the policy process relating to palliative care planning and provision, and to suggest avenues for evaluation research.

Practical evaluation: opportunities and constraints

Evaluation is purposeful, applied research, undertaken to solve practical problems; and it is important that it should be recognized as being embedded in a wider context. Evaluation is particularly important because of the fiscal pressures on health care systems, which have intensified since the 1980s. Unless society is content to be taxed ever more to finance the increasing health care bill, or to pay ever higher insurance premiums, or to pay increased amounts 'out of pocket', then decisions have to be made about the fairest and most cost-effective manner to allocate resources between competing health care sectors. Pressures for evaluation come therefore from a complex political context, and it is important to understand the existence of multiple stakeholders in any evaluation, and to take account of their visible or hidden roles. But who are the stakeholders in relation to evaluation research in palliative care? The following list suggests the more obvious candidates (adapted from Rossi and Freeman, 1993).

Stakeholders in palliative care

Type of stakeholder

Policy and decision makers	Government (at different levels) Professional groups (medical, nursing, social work, other therapists) National advisory and consultative groups (and pressure groups)
Service funders or sponsors	Health and social service commissioning and funding agencies at the district, regional, and national level Charitable bodies
Evaluation funders or sponsors	Research councils Health service commissioners Charitable bodies Palliative care service providers
Service target participants	Patients Family carers and friends Health professionals
Service management	Hospice and palliative care team managers Hospital managers Community or primary care managers
Service staff	Health care professionals Social workers and other non-clinical professionals Administrative, secretarial, domestic, and other support staff Volunteers
Evaluators	University or freelance 'outside' researchers Members of staff of the palliative care service
Service competitors / collaborators	Other palliative care services in the vicinity Other non-palliative care specialties in the vicinity

Contextual stakeholders	Society
	Carer / user networks
	Interest groups
Evaluation community	Other research groups involved in palliative care evaluation
	Other groups of health service or clinical researchers

This is quite an impressive list, and it is probably not exhaustive. An evaluation will not need to negotiate with all the stakeholders mentioned above, but it is a salutary reminder that there is a great potential for research to have a wide impact. Too often this potential is not realized, either because evaluations fizzle out, or they were misconceived and get put aside, or their results fail to get disseminated in an effective way. As well, a problem that can arise is that conflicts in the interests of these stakeholders can put a strain on the integrity of the evaluation. Evaluators will sometimes have to cope with these conflicts, and may be undecided as to whose perspective to take, or whose to give priority to. It is a skill to be able to communicate with different stakeholders in ways which lessen their misunderstandings of the work and, thus, the chance of the research being rejected, or worse, being ridiculed. Being the subject of an evaluation is not always a pleasant experience and evaluators, especially if they come from outside the service or organization being evaluated, do face the possibility of resentment, secrecy, and obstruction. This is particularly so if the aims and methods of the evaluation have not been clarified, or understood, and if the data collection methods are regarded as burdensome, intrusive, or unethical.

Who should evaluate palliative care?

The evaluator can be regarded as a stakeholder in the evaluation, partly because he or she may represent a particular organization or position, and also because many decisions will be taken during the research process which will be idiosyncratic, and may even reflect personal opinion. To date, much of the research in the field of palliative care has been carried out by researchers working in universities who have developed a personal interest in the subject, and by practitioners working in either academic departments with palliative care teams or in the larger, more well-established hospices.

In relation to the status of the evaluator of the organization or service, there are several points to be made. There is little reason for a categorical preference for either internal or external evaluation. Evaluators are diverse in their activities and working arrangements, and what might be gained by impartiality and neutrality (outsider) might be offset by the lack of knowledge of processes and under-standing of the context (insider). What is crucial is that evalu-ators have a clear understanding of their role in a given situation. In the case of service practitioners, this may involve adopting a more critical and disinterested approach to their clinical work, and also persuading their colleagues that they are to be trusted with in-formation not normally made available. These points only serve to emphasize the need for evaluators to understand their own role, and to negotiate entry to the research situation in an appropriate manner.

Timing and timeliness of evaluations

Both the timing and timeliness of evaluations are important con-siderations that can make the difference between success or failure. Robson suggests that 'evaluations are things to avoid unless you have a good chance of doing them properly' (Robson 1993). He considers that there is no point in doing an evaluation unless it is going to be useful to someone; unless it can be carried out with technical skill and sensitivity, unless it can be carried out fairly and ethically; and unless it is feasible to conduct it in practical terms. However, there are various pressures which are liable to distort all of these good intentions. One pressure comes from the mismatch between political time and evaluation time. Because evaluations are done for a purpose, a number of decisions may be hanging on the results. Evaluators of a new service or demonstration project will be under pressure to report so that decisions relating to the next year's funding can be made—which could involve jobs, new premises, or a number of developments that require forward planning. However, research that is unduly hurried, prematurely completed, or reduced in scale is likely to produce unreliable results; thus wasting the evaluation funds, the energies of the evaluator, and possibly jeopardising his or her credibility. At the start of an evaluation, it is therefore important to negotiate the time-scale—to ensure a balance between the needs of the organization and the integrity of the research design.

A related point concerns the timeliness of the evaluation. For some evaluations, particularly those funded by research councils or other national grant-awarding bodies, there can be a lengthy lead-in to the research. The process of applying for funds and acquiring all necessary permissions for the work (particularly if multiple sites are involved) lengthens the time from the identification of the need for the evaluation to when the research actually starts. By the time the research has finished and the recommendations have been made it is conceivable that the world has moved on, and the questions have changed. This is of course a danger in all research, but it is particularly unfortunate in evaluation research which is only really worthwhile if the results are used.

Dissemination

Evaluators need to put a high priority on deliberately planning for the dissemination of the results of their work, and they need to be able to package the findings in ways that are geared to the requirements and competencies of a range of relevant stakeholders. Evaluations which have been carried out with research council funds, and by outside researchers, are more likely to be reported in a range of specialist and non-specialist journals, and perhaps even in the popular media. Evaluations carried out 'in-house' will probably be reported in internal documents with restricted readership. Whatever the style of dissemination, it should be in a form that encourages the understanding of the results and any recommendations for changing practice.

It has been recognized that it is notoriously difficult to change clinical practice even in the face of reliable and valid evidence. Despite efficient and targeted dissemination of results, it is still possible that evidence from some forms of evaluation will have little impact. Increasingly, researchers are encouraging the adoption of collaborative forms of evaluation, which engage the various relevant stakeholders in the process, thereby increasing the chances that findings, which are meaningful to the stakeholders, are more likely to be acted upon (Everitt and Hardiker 1996).

Policy and decision making in palliative care: can evaluation help?

Specialist palliative care services have developed rapidly in the UK and elsewhere, in a relatively unco-ordinated manner. In the UK, there has been a general absence of clear national policy relating to what sort of palliative care should be provided, in what settings, and out of which budget. Guidance from the National Health Service Executive to district health service commissioners has tended to be supportive of the aims of specialist palliative care, and of the voluntary hospice sector, although voluntary providers are expected to bid for their NHS funds in line with other health care providers. The development of strategic palliative care purchasing at the district level may well have been hindered by the *ad hoc* development of a buoyant voluntary sector, and the lack of national policy.

Policy formation

Since the early 1990s, attempts have been made to formulate policy in relation to palliative care provision. The NCHSPCS has been particularly important in this respect, as have some of the national cancer charities in their lobbying capacity (for example, Cancer Relief Macmillan Fund and Marie Curie Cancer Care). The Standing Medical Advisory Committee and Standing Nursing and Midwifery Advisory Committee made a series of recommendations in 1992 about the principles and provision of palliative care. Importantly, their report recommended that services should not be limited to patients with cancer. As a result of these recommendations (or coincidentally) many hospices have widened their admission criteria, and Marie Curie Cancer Care now offers its home care nurses to patients of all diagnoses—although they only reimburse the costs of nursing care (up to 50 per cent) for the patients suffering from cancer. Another important policy document is the report of the Expert Advisory Group on Cancer to the Chief Medical Officers of England and Wales (1995)—popularly known as the Calman Hine Report—which proposes a network of cancer care services in England and Wales. The implementation of this 'strategic framework' is under way at the time of writing, and so it is impossible to draw conclusions as to its likely impact. Although primary care is seen as the focus of care, there are recommendations regarding the input of specialist palliative care in the designated cancer units and cancer centres. In relation to palliative care, item 4.5.2 states that 'each district must have a specialist resource for both primary care and hospital based services' (Expert Advisory Group on Cancer to the Chief Medical Officers of England and Wales 1995).

While these suggested frameworks can be seen as the first faltering steps towards a comprehensive national policy for palliative care, it could be argued that full policy formation is still some way off. Banting (1979) suggests that there are five stages in policy formation: awareness of the problem; the important or salience of the problem; definition of the problem; specification of alternatives; and finally, the choice between alternatives. If these five stages are applied to the problem of palliative care provision, then it can be seen that not all requirements are met:

1. *Awareness of the problem*
Awareness of the 'distress of dying' arose during the 1950s and 60s. The opening of St Christopher's Hospice in 1967 was instrumental in raising general awareness that there were the effective means to address the palliative care needs of the terminally ill.

2. *Importance of the problem*
Since the 1970s, surveys have demonstrated the severity of uncontrolled symptoms and psychosocial distress amongst cancer patients in hospital and community settings. Recently, the palliative care needs of patients with non-cancer diagnoses have been identified and given prominence.

3. *Definition of the problem*
Assessing the palliative care needs of populations (as opposed to individuals) is difficult, partly because there has been confusion about the definition of palliative care (hospice, specialist, specialty, and so on), and how it differs to mainstream / conventional care (and whether it should differ). The NCHSPCS (1995*a*) has issued a statement of definitions which attempts to bring clarity to this.

4. *Specification of alternatives*
Palliative care is provided in a range of settings, sometimes replacing, and sometimes supplementing standard clinical care. It is not clear what the most effective and appropriate care alternatives or options are. There is a marked lack of evidence regarding the quality, cost, and feasibility of alternative models of palliative care.

5. Choice between alternatives

At present, the evidence base is insufficient to choose between alternative forms of palliative care provision, or to choose the most effective mix of types of provision.

An important feature of palliative care provision to bear in mind is the involvement of the charitable/voluntary sector. Charitably-funded specialist palliative care services have developed within a long tradition in the UK of the pioneering and gap-filling role of voluntary organizations *vis-à-vis* statutory services (Lewis 1994). Many hospice services have developed to the point they have partly because of a confused ideology about what the NHS should provide, what it can afford, what the public demand of it, and what the public regard as 'optional extras'. There is charitable input in many areas of health care—blood donation, refreshment outlets in hospitals, fund-raising to provide equipment or to fund medical research, and so on. These activities can be labelled very broadly as supportive, and are seldom questioned. However, when charitable input provides substantial amounts of direct patient care, as in the case of many specialist palliative care services, then it is less clear how they stand in relation to the planning and commissioning functions of the statutory services. The formation of national and district policy may even be subverted by the independence of a voluntary sector of provision which, once up and running, develops an internal momentum to keep running and even expand. While the voluntary sector of palliative care has facilitated tremendous innovation and dissemination of good practice, as well as delivering highly valued services to countless patients and their families, it also acts to deflect attention away from developing fully-funded statutory provision.

The stages of policy formation as outlined are useful for debating the various strengths and weaknesses of the different models of palliative care. A priority for policy and decision makers must be to reach the stage where national policy can be formulated, and then to examine the ways in which the policy can be most successfully implemented. However, the present lack of relevant evidence provides a clear role for evaluation research to furnish the appropriate evidence for feeding into the policy formation process.

A framework for evaluation

The evidence presented in this book has demonstrated that researchers have faced difficulties in carrying out evaluations of palliative care, particularly at the level of service effectiveness. People who are terminally ill obviously present a research challenge; not only do there have to be adequate safeguards within any research design to protect patients from undue harassment and invasion of their privacy, but the nature of the patient group can be distressing to the researchers themselves. However, specialist services have developed to address the particular needs and concerns of the terminally ill, and it is right that such services should be evaluated for their efficiency, effectiveness, and appropriateness. This section discusses three aspects of palliative care evaluation: setting appropriate outcome indicators; adopting appropriate research designs; and making feasible comparisons. There are suggestions for ways in which these methods and perspectives can be set to work.

Performance indicators and outcome measures   Studies discussed in the preceding chapter have suggested a range of performance indicators and outcome measures which are relevant to palliative care. Because the objectives of palliative care are different to those of curative clinical care, outcome indicators need to reflect the changed priorities over patient care, and the enhanced weight given to quality of life factors. Tables 6.1–6.4 attempt to map a range of outcome indicators that could be used in the assessment of palliative care. (Patient-based outcomes of course depend on patients being able to fill in questionnaires and answer questions, and many will not be able to do this at varying times during the terminal illness.) In addition to these performance and outcome indicators, which can be used to describe both the process and outcome of palliative care, there are a range of subjective or qualitative factors which are more difficult to codify and define. They include things like 'atmosphere', 'attitude', 'busyness', and of course 'personality'. The question of the *time* available to care for patients with terminal illness is also important, and only partially measured through workload data. Inpatient hospices have higher staff to patient ratios than other institutional settings, and home care nurses have lower workloads than community nurses. Tierney *et al.* found that staff in an independent hospice spent more time on direct patient care than staff

Table 6.1 Patient-based outcome indicators in palliative care

Patient-based outcomes	Methods of assessment	Comments
Control/severity of symptoms	Structured self-complete symptom checklists	Widely used method. Some instruments produce an overall score which can be useful for demonstrating differences between patient groups
	Patient-generated symptom checklists (with or without Visual Analogue Score or weighting procedure)	Increasingly being used in addition to structured instruments. Best used to chart individual change in symptom burden over time.
Quality of life	Structured self-complete instruments or self evaluations (e.g. SEIQoL)	Wide selection of validated instruments mostly developed in oncology setting. Limited in their sensitivity to changes in meaning of life. Instruments being developed for use in palliative care.
Satisfaction with location of care, speed and nature of response of health and social care professionals (including communication)	Questionnaires and interview	Patients may not be able to comment critically on the care they are receiving, nor to compare it with other possible models of care.

Table 6.2 Home carer-based outcome indicators in palliative care

Home carer-based outcomes	Methods of assessment	Comments
Satisfaction with care given to patient and with care and support (practical help) given to home carer (including communication)	Questionnaires (e.g. FAMCARE) and interviews	Can be done prospectively and retrospectively (possibility of recall bias), and can indicate gaps in service provision
Household costs (financial and social) associated with terminal illness	Diaries and detailed questionnaires during time of terminal illness	Can only be done accurately prospectively. Only possible with home carers who can cope with method
Risk of severe grief reaction	Structured measures of psychological morbidity (e.g. HADS). Risk assessment scores	Intensity of the grief reaction may be unrelated to the quality of the services given during terminal illness
Satisfaction with bereavement support	Questionnaires and interviews	Might need to be combined with risk score. Time intervals might need to be comparable

Table 6.3 Staff-based outcome indicators in palliative care

Staff-based outcomes	Methods of assessment	Comments
Satisfaction with nature of care delivered	Questionnaires (e.g. STAS) and interviews	May be biased since staff are being asked to assess their own performance
Efficiency of communication between different professionals	Telephone interviews, checklists, questionnaires	Important for highlighting gaps in communication, could be carried out as an audit exercise
Speed of response to requests for help	Audit of records e.g. time between referral to services and take-up	Can be used for assessing service efficiency
Levels of work-related stress	Self-complete measures of psychological morbidity, interviews	Useful to compare the experiences of staff working in different settings and with different amounts of team support
Satisfaction with working environment, clinical supervision, and staff support procedures	Records of staff turnover and absences, questionnaires, interviews, focus group discussions	Important for assessing levels of staff morale
Access to training, education, study leave, conferences, etc.	Data from staff records combined with questionnaires	Needs to be linked in with availability of courses and amount of funding available. Also needs evidence of short and long-term outcome.

Table 6.4 Service-based outcome indicators in palliative care

Service-based outcomes	Methods of assessment	Comments
Utilization of services	Routine activity data	Relies on accurate, up-to-date, and complete records. Many hospices need to review their record-keeping procedures. Linkage between datasets gives better picture of use of services
Staff workload and staffing levels	Staff rotas and case-load figures	Important for comparisons between different providers. High case-load levels are not necessarily indications of efficiency in palliative care
Perceptions of different service providers of quality of services	Questionnaires, focus group discussions	Planners and purchasers should be involved with providers in negotiating best models of care
Place of death	Mortality data	Impact of services can be tracked using place of death as a marker
Costs of different types of care	Accounts from hospices, specialist teams, nursing homes, and other providers, with additional prescribing data where possible	Very difficult to compare costs, but basic hotel and care costs should be available for the different inpatient settings

in an NHS hospice, implying that pressures across the NHS work to reduce patient contact time (Tierney *et al.* 1994)—although, of course, 'time' is not by itself an indicator of the quality of care.

Research design   As a result of over 40 years of work in the field of programme evaluation in the United States, Cronbach wrote in 1982 that 'Evaluation is an art' and that 'there is no single best plan for an evaluation, not even for an inquiry into a particular program, at a particular time, with a particular budget'. (Cronbach 1982). Cronbach's conclusions suggest that there is little room for methodological dogmatism in the field of evaluation. In relation to palliative care research, a wide range of research methods have been used, some to better effect than others. Experimental methods have been harder to apply at the service level, while cross-sectional, retrospective surveys of satisfaction have been found to be of use for service planning.

Feasible comparisons   The most appropriate research design to be used in an evaluation will depend on the question being asked. However, evaluation depends on comparison, and Table 6.5 suggests the types of research design that can be used for making a number of different comparisons. The emphasis of Table 6.5 is on *service* evaluation, since this is the type of evaluation that will best feed into policymaking. Specific palliative care interventions and therapies of course require testing for their safety, acceptability, iatrogenic effect, and so on, but a collection of efficacious and effective therapies does not necessarily produce an effective service. There are some comparisons that are very difficult to make, particularly those that involve hospice services. Because there is no automatic referral to hospice services, and patients do have preferences about accepting hospice input, it is questionable whether under current practice an experimental design could address the matter of the effectiveness of hospice care in relation to non-hospice care. Experimental designs are complex in the other contexts mentioned, but they do have the capacity to produce comparative data from groups that are similar in every respect except for the receipt of the palliative care service. Although surveys have shown that patients' home carers are more satisfied with the care they receive from palliative care services than from conventional services (Cartwright and Seale 1990; Dawson 1991; Wakefield and Ashby

Table 6.5 Types of research design for use for making different comparisons

Level of evaluation	Type of comparison	Feasible research design
Within single palliative care service	Comparison of actual practice with goals (aims and objectives)	Case-study approach involving the analysis of service policies and aims, an examination of practice, and an examination of the effects
	Comparison of service before a change in practice (or context) and afterwards	Longitudinal study (using survey design)
		Possible natural experiment if not all parts of the service are affected by the change, and if baseline data can be collected before change happens
Between different palliative care services	Comparison of service characteristics	Cross-sectional survey. Useful for descriptive purposes but unable to make causal associations between types of care and apparent outcomes
		Case-studies. Will generate in-depth contextual data, possibly useful for theory generalizability
		Randomized controlled trial. This could be difficult because patient choice is likely to be important, preventing random allocation to groups. A preference trial of hospice at home versus inpatient hospice care might be feasible
Between palliative care service and standard care without palliative care service	Comparison of effectiveness, cost, and preference	Matched comparison study (controlled trial). Difficult to draw conclusions unless sophisticated modelling of the threats to validity
		Randomized controlled trial. This might be possible where patients are cared for in a setting where specialist and non-specialist care is provided, e.g. in a hospital with a palliative care team service, or in the community with a palliative home care team service
		Case-studies. As above

1993), the association between satisfaction and care received is confounded by a number of home carer related variables. Studies that have shown superiority in process aspects of palliative care in comparison to conventional care are persuasive—for example, communication is more open under palliative care (Centeno-Cortés and Núñez-Olarte 1994), care goals are set quicker (Lunt and Neale 1987), and non-specialists highly rate the input of specialists (see Table 4.2, pp. 98–9)—however, these studies do not provide evidence of impact on patient outcomes.

Because of the vulnerability and frailty of the palliative care population, the choice of research design is not easy. Understanding the advantages of experimental approaches and using them when possible is important. At the same time, it must be accepted that the definition of 'evidence' needs to be inclusive enough to embrace the findings of all research, as long as it has been carried out systematically, rigorously, and with attention to modelling the threats to its validity.

Needs' assessment evaluation

This final section attempts to locate the evaluation strategies and perspectives just described back into the real world of palliative care. A recurring theme throughout these chapters has been the need for palliative care, and the matching up of that need with appropriate services. Clearly, and rationally, the first step in assessing the need for palliative care is the evaluation of best models of palliative care provision as described. If the effectiveness of different types of care is unknown, then of course it is difficult to estimate the numbers in the population who might require those service *and benefit from them*. It is possible to see how the following model of needs' assessment could be applied (after Frankel 1991):

(1) the distribution in the population of those for whom specialist palliative care is indicated and desired;

(2) the effectiveness of specialist palliative care for specified categories of person;

(3) justification in terms of benefits per unit cost that the care of such cases is an appropriate investment in relation to competing services.

This model requires evidence of the effectiveness of palliative care services for specified categories of person, and then of the distribution in the population of those persons for whom those palliative care services are indicated and desired (Higginson 1997). Finally, some kind of resource allocation criteria are needed to establish that spending limited health care funds on this kind of care brings a large enough 'health gain' for it to be justified (taking into account all the other patient care demands in other specialties and sectors).

The rationality of this model cannot be denied, but its application to palliative care appears tenuous. Part of the difficulty is the inability to place fences around what is palliative care and what is not. As an example of this, Fig. 6.1 suggests how varied and complex the experience of inpatient care may be. (This discussion focuses on the situation in the UK, and it is acknowledged that there will be similarities and differences to other countries.) This complex mosaic of services will itself be affected by variables operating in the local context which can obfuscate both the assessment of effectiveness and the indications for such effective service provision. These areas of variability are shown in Table 6.6.It can be seen that palliative care

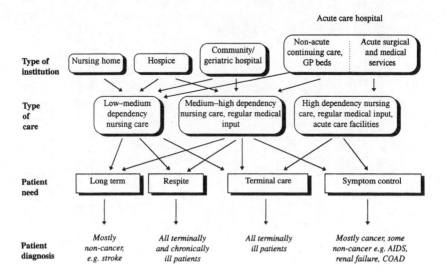

Figure 6.1   Web of need, provision, and care for patients requiring inpatient admissions

Table 6.6 Sources of variability in the assessment of need for palliative care services

Service level	Population level	Patient level	Clinician level
Characteristics of local health services, e.g. availability of acute and non-acute care beds in different types of institution, availability of 24-hour community support	Demographic profile of population and availability of home carers	Type of terminal illness according to diagnosis and site	Patterns of hospital and community follow-up for patients with terminal illness
Characteristics of tertiary referral services, e.g. follow-up services from oncology centres	Socio-economic and cultural profile of population	Severity of symptoms and psychosocial problems	Existing levels of competency in palliative care and availability of local training
Characteristics of local specialist palliative care services, e.g. models of nursing care, availability of inpatient hospice beds, provision of hospice at home service	Geographical spread of population (urban/rural)	Availability of social support	Attitude to collaboration with specialist and voluntary palliative care services
Levels of local funding for health and social services and national policy	Local support for voluntary services	Preferences regarding location of care, including attitude to hospice care	Local budgeting/management arrangements

services are already organized and delivered against a complex background of service, population, patient, and clinician variables, and taking all of these into account at any one time is problematic.

Population requiring palliative care The question of how many people within a health care district are likely to require palliative care services over a set period depends on the indications for specialist intervention. Because the remit of palliative care services is wide, so the indications for palliative care are also wide. Difficulties with symptom management and/or hindrances within the family or home situation requiring more input than either community nurses or GPs can provide, may prompt referrals to palliative care services. That is, the problems are severe enough to necessitate specialist help. Alternatively, palliative care services may be involved as a matter of routine in almost all cases of terminal cancer illness, and their input will vary according to the level of patient need.

The need for community-based palliative care support centres around routine nursing procedures which can be carried out in the home, respite nursing or sitting services to allow the home carer, (if there is one) to catch up on sleep or go out, emotional support for the patient and the home carer and the provision of information as well as help over access to equipment and aids (such as special mattresses, hoists, or syringe drivers). Both palliative care providers and the NHS community nursing services aim to meet all the needs already described, although the specialist nurses are less likely to carry out 'hands-on' care (as discussed in Chapter 4). Intensive home care nursing services (24-hour care) can be provided from both sources in some areas. Equipment can be supplied by the community nursing services through their own NHS equipment supplies, but they also arrange loans from the Red Cross who keep a range of aids and equipment for use during terminal illness. The overlap between specialist services and routine services in the community setting is potentially considerable. However, specialist palliative care nurses do have more time at their disposal to spend with patients, with workloads about a quarter of the size of those of community nurses (Robbins and Frankel 1995).

In the hospital setting, the need for palliative care support springs from the inability of other hospital clinicians to meet the psychosocial and symptom control needs of inpatients. What specialist palliative care services might offer are staff who could spend more time with patients and their families than the ward staff, education and training to non-specialists in psychosocial counselling skills, and physical symptom control advice. They could also help co-ordinate the discharge and follow-up of the patient with the primary health care team.

Most formal assessments of the need for specialist palliative care services have focused on the need for inpatient provision. Although Lunt and Hillier concluded their review of hospice services in 1980 with the recommendation that home care and hospital support teams should be developed, rather than inpatient units, they suggested that 40–50 palliative care beds per million population seemed an adequate level of inpatient provision (Lunt and Hillier 1981). They observed that hospital support teams might reduce this requirement by improving the control of symptoms in existing hospitals. This figure was corroborated by other researchers planning services in health districts which had no inpatient palliative care beds. For example, Frankel and Kammerling's assessment of the need for hospice beds in one health district—using both routine statistics that describe the general pattern of deaths, and also a survey of relevant practitioners' likely referral rates had such an inpatient unit existed—similarly concluded that a figure of around 50 beds per million population was a reasonable guide (Frankel and Kammerling 1990). However, having monitored the first year's activity data, and also taking into account their original estimates, Frankel and Kammerling caution that the population denominator has to take into account effective access to a proposed hospice. Many health districts have topological or historical features which demarcate lines of communication within the population, and these can affect the actual patterns of service usage.

Calculations of the requirement for inpatient palliative care have tended to concentrate on people with a diagnosis of cancer, and it is recognized that assessing the need for specialist palliative care for the wider population of cancer and non-cancer patients is more difficult. Wilson *et al.* (1995) attempted to assess the need for inpatient palliative care facilities for non-cancer patients in three health districts in central southern England and showed that current levels of provision would have to be tripled to accommodate the needs for respite and continuing palliative care of these people. However, this study demonstrates how difficult it is to calculate the effect of extending hospice-type provision to incorporate the psychogeriatric care, and stroke rehabilitation required by many of the non-cancer patients. Such patients have a different range of clinical needs, but their social needs for respite care (day care and planned inpatient admissions) and community support may be similar to patients with cancer. (This convergent need is portrayed in Fig. 6.1.)

Assessments of the need for palliative care in other settings have also been carried out. Some of these studies have taken a district or regional view (Zalot 1989; Partridge 1989; Downing *et al.* 1993), while others have focused on the need for palliative care support within the hospital setting and how it can be organized (Simpson 1976; Severs and Wilkins 1991; James *et al.* 1985; Barrelet and Caillet Jousson 1993; Bircumshaw 1993). The study of James *et al.* in Australia concluded that between five and ten per cent of all patients in large teaching hospitals may be so ill that they have a likely prognosis of around three months, implying that palliative care services should be able to cater for up to 10 per cent of the total hospital inpatient population at any one time (James *et al.* 1985). However, it is not clear exactly what form hospital palliative care services should take. Should the service have designated beds to recreate a hospice-type ward within the hospital, like that proposed by Severs and Wilkins (1991), or should it consist of a team of staff who integrate their care with that already being offered to patients (for example, the psychosocial counselling team for AIDS patients described by Barnes *et al.* 1993)? To what extent should hospital-based palliative care teams offer domiciliary follow-up and how does this then affect the assessment of need for community-based specialist palliative care nurses? At present there are no obvious answers to these questions, and it does not seem to be clear either, what the 'right' level of community-based specialist palliative care nursing input should be. As the study of Eve and Smith (1994) reveals, there is tremendous variability in the level and volume of services, but what is unknown is exactly what the level *should be*. Responding to patient demand is of course one way of setting a level that is appropriate in a local context, although it is well-known that patient demand is itself sensitive to a range of extraneous pressures.

While not rejecting the rationality of the needs' assessment model, it is clear that the heterogeneity of palliative care services complicates the application of the model. This is the 'real world' of palliative care research; neither a neat nor tidy set of practices to evaluate.

Concluding remarks

This chapter has drawn attention to the gaps in the evidence base of palliative care, and also attempted to provide some pointers to the kind of work that is required in the future. The development of a strong, independent research programme in palliative care is important for a number of reasons. As a complicated package of care that crosses boundaries between social and health care, and primary and secondary care, and where utility measures based on quantity of survival time are clearly inappropriate, the methodological challenges of research in palliative care are particularly pressing. In particular, methods of assessing the requirement for palliative care on the basis of symptomatology, nursing need, domestic circumstances, and psychosocial need, have to be developed, as do methods which are able to model the time-dependent nature of the changing needs of the terminally ill population.

The necessity to develop palliative care research has been recognized for many years in the face of the rapid expansion of services, and considerable progress has already been achieved. However, the next few years will see increasing pressure for the palliative care sector to justify its 'anecdotal success and emotional appeal' (Lunt and Hillier 1981). In a sea of change, rippling with performance indicators, total quality management, patient charters, public accountability, and fear of litigation, the concept of evaluation is politically apt. No sector—public, private, or voluntary—can afford to ignore the assertions of those who maintain that if health care is not seen to be based on 'good' evidence of its effectiveness then it is not worth paying for.

At the end of the day, dying is often a sad and distressing time for all concerned and palliative care does not change that. Palliative care can help to anaesthetize the pain of the biological death, facilitate acceptance of the void of the social death, and offer company to the individual in his or her quest for the philosophical, existential, or spiritual meaning of death. This book has offered an introduction to the evaluation of this field of care and the complexities involved. It has posed more questions than it has answered, and it has attempted to expose the difficulties in dissecting the concept of effectiveness by looking in turn at the perspectives of the various interested parties. It is hoped that in its own way, this book will help to advance a sophisticated and rigorous approach to palliative care evaluation.

References

Aaronson, N.K., *et al.* (1993). The European Organization for Research and Treatment of Cancer QLQ-C30: a quality of life instrument for use in international clinical trials in oncology. *Journal of the National Cancer Institute*, **85**, 365–76.

Addington-Hall, J.M., MacDonald, L.D., Anderson, H.R., and Freeling, P. (1991). Dying from cancer: the views of bereaved family and friends about the experiences of terminally ill patients. *Palliative Medicine*, **5**, 207–14.

Addington-Hall, J.M., *et al.* (1992). Randomised controlled trial of effects of coordinating care for terminally ill cancer patients. *British Medical Journal*, **305**, 1317–22.

Addington-Hall, J. and McCarthy, M. (1995). Regional study of care for the dying: methods and sample characteristics. *Palliative Medicine*, **9**, 27–35.

Ajemian, I. (1993*a*). The interdisciplinary team. In *Oxford textbook of palliative medicine* (ed. D. Doyle, G. Hanks, and N. MacDonald), pp. 17–27. Oxford University Press.

Ajemian, I. (1993*b*). Training of volunteers in palliative care. In *Oxford textbook of palliative medicine* (ed. D. Doyle, G. Hanks, and N. Mac-Donald), pp. 799–801. Oxford University Press.

Alexander, D.A. and Ritchie, E. (1990). 'Stressors' and difficulties in dealing with the terminal patient. *Journal of Palliative Care*, **6**, 28–33.

Alexander, D.A. and MacLeod, M. (1992). Stress among palliative care matrons: a major problem for a minority group. *Palliative Medicine*, **6**, 111–24.

Alexander, D.A. (1993). Staff support groups: do they support and are they even groups? *Palliative Medicine*, **7**, 127–32.

Anderson, F., Downing, G.M., Hill, J., Casorso, L., and Lerch, N. (1996). Palliative Performance Scale (PPS): a new tool. *Journal of Palliative Care*, **12**, 5–11.

Anonymous. (1983). Cancer care: the relative's view. *Lancet*, **ii**, 1188–9.

Appleton, R., Gibson, B., and Hey, E. (1993). The loss of a baby at birth: the role of the bereavement officer. *British Journal of Obstetrics and Gynaecology*, **100**, 51–4.

Ashley, J. and Devis, T. (1992). Death certification from the point of view of the epidemiologist. In *OPCS, population trends, spring 1992*, (pp. 22–8).

Athlin, E., Furåker, C., Jansson, L., and Norberg, A. (1993). Application of primary nursing within a team setting in the hospice care of cancer patients. *Cancer Nursing*, **16**, 388–97.

Banting, K. (1979). *Poverty, politics and policy*. Macmillan, London.

Barnes, R., Barrett, C., Weintraub, S., Holowacz, G., Chan, M., and Leblanc, E. (1993). Hospital response to psychosocial needs of AIDS inpatients. *Journal of Palliative Care*, 9, 22–8.

Barrelet, L. and Caillet Jousson, A-M. (1993). Organization of palliative care in a general hospital. *Palliative Medicine*, 7 (suppl. 1), 39–43.

Barritt, P.W. (1984). Care of the dying in one practice. *Journal of the Royal College of General Practitioners*, 34, 446–8.

Bartley, M. (1985). Coronary heart disease and the public health 1850–1983. *Sociology of Health and Illness*, 7, 289–313.

Bates, T., Hoy, A.M., Clarke, D.G., and Laird, P.P. (1981). The St Thomas' hospital terminal care support team. *Lancet*, May 30, 1201–3.

Bennett, M. and Corcoran, G. (1994). The impact on community palliative care services of a hospital palliative care team. *Palliative Medicine*, 8, 237–44.

Bernard, H.R. (1988). *Research methods in cultural anthropology.* Sage, California.

Berterö, C. and Ek, A-C. (1993). Quality of life of adults with acute leukaemia. *Journal of Advanced Nursing*, 18, 1346–53.

Bircumshaw, D. (1993). Palliative care in the acute hospital setting. *Journal of Advanced Nursing*, 18, 1665–6.

Bloor, M.J., Robertson, C., and Samphier, M.L. (1989). Occupational status variations in disagreements on the diagnosis of cause of death. *Human Pathology*, 20, 144–8.

Bowling, A. (1995). *Measuring disease*, p. 2. Open University Press, Buckingham.

Boyd, K.J. (1992). The working patterns of hospice based home care teams. *Palliative Medicine*, 6, 131–9.

Boyd, K.J. (1993). Palliative care in the community: views of general practitioners and district nurses in East London. *Journal of Palliative Care*, 9, 33–7.

Boyd, K.J. (1995). The role of specialist home care teams: views of general practitioners in south London. *Palliative Medicine*, 9, 138–44.

Bradshaw, P.J. (1993). Characteristics of clients referred to home, hospice and hospital palliative care services in Western Australia. *Palliative Medicine*, 7, 101–7.

Bromberg, M.H. and Higginson, I. (1996). Bereavement follow-up: what do palliative support teams actually do? *Journal of Palliative Care*, 12, 12–17.

Brooks, C.H. and Smyth-Staruch, K. (1984). Hospice home care cost-savings to third-party insurers. *Medical Care*, 22, 691–703.

Brooks, R. (1995). *Health status measurement: a perspective on change.* Macmillan, Basingstoke.

Bruera, E. and MacDonald, S. (1993). Audit methods: The Edmonton Symptom Assessment System. In *Clinical audit in palliative care* (ed. I. Higginson), pp. 61–77. Radcliffe Medical Press, Oxford.

Bruera, E. (1994). Ethical issues in palliative care research. *Journal of Palliative Care*, **10**, 7–9.

Bryant, A. and Payne, S. (1993). Difficulties inherent in research with cancer patients. *Journal of Cancer Care*, **2**, 143–6.

Bryman, A. and Burgess, R.G. (1994). Reflections on qualitative data analysis. In *Analyzing qualitative data* (ed. A. Bryman and R.G. Burgess), pp. 216–26. Routledge, London.

Butler, D. (1994). Palliative care in general practice—a new initiative. European *Journal of Palliative Care*, **1**, 8–10.

Butters, E., Higginson, I., George, R., and McCarthy, M. (1993). Palliative care for people with HIV/AIDS: views of patients, carers and providers. *AIDS Care*, **5**, 105–16.

Buxton, M. and Hanney, S. (1996). How can payback from health services research be assessed? *Journal of Health Services Research and Policy*, **1**, 35–43.

Calman, K.C. and Hanks, G. (1993). Clinical and health services research in palliative care. In *Oxford textbook of palliative medicine* (ed. D. Doyle, G. Hanks, and N. MacDonald), pp. 73–7. Oxford University Press.

Carey, J.W. (1993). Linking qualitative and quantitative methods: integrating cultural factors into public health. *Qualitative Health Research*, **3**, 298–318.

Cartwright, A. and Seale, C. (1990). *The natural history of a survey: an account of the methodological issues encountered in a study of life before death*. King Edward's Hospital Fund for London.

Cassel, C.K. and Vladeck, B.C. (1996). ICD-9 Code for palliative or terminal care. *New England Journal of Medicine*, **335**, 1232–4.

Cawley, N. and Webber, J. (1995). Research priorities in palliative care. *International Journal of Palliative Nursing*, **1**, 101–13.

Cawley, N. (1997). An exploration of the concept of spirituality. *International Journal of Palliative Nursing*, **3**, 31–6.

Centeno-Cortés, C. and Núñez-Olarte, J. (1994). Questioning diagnosis disclosure in terminal cancer patients: a prospective study evaluating patients' responses. *Palliative Medicine*, **8**, 39–44.

Chen, H-T. (1988). Validity in evaluation research: a critical assessment of current issues. *Policy and Politics*, **16**, 1–16.

Choinière, M. and Amsel, R. (1996). A visual analogue thermometer for measuring pain intensity. *Journal of Pain and Symptom Management*, **11**, 299–311.

Clark, D. (1993*a*). Whither the hospices? In *The future for palliative care* (ed. D. Clark), pp. 167–77. Open University Press, Buckingham.

Clark, D. (1993*b*). Evaluating the needs of informal carers. *Progress in Palliative Care*, **1**, 3–5.

Clark, D. (1997). What is qualitative research and what can it contribute to palliative care? *Palliative Medicine*, **11**, 159–166.

Clark, P. and Bowling A. (1990). Quality of everyday life in long-stay institutions for the elderly. An observational study of long-stay hospital and nursing home care. *Social Science and Medicine*, **30**, 1201–10.

Clein, P. (1997). Local research ethics committees in the UK. *Palliative Medicine*, **11**, 55–6.

Clinch, J.R. and Schipper, H. (1993). Quality of life assessment in palliative care. In *Oxford textbook of palliative medicine* (ed. D. Doyle, G. Hanks, and N. MacDonald), pp. 61–70. Oxford University Press.

Cohen, S.R., Mount, B., Strobel, M.G., and Bui, F. (1995). The McGill Quality of Life Questionnaire: a measure of quality of life appropriate for people with advanced disease. A preliminary study of validity and acceptability. *Palliative Medicine*, **9**, 207–19.

Cohen, S.R., Mount, B.M., Bruera, E., Provost, M., Rowe, J., and Tong, K. (1997). Validity of the McGill Quality of Life Questionnaire in the palliative care setting: a multi-centre Canadian study demonstrating the importance of the existential domain. *Palliative Medicine*, **11**, 3–20.

Coles, C. (1996). Undergraduate education and palliative care. *Palliative Medicine*, **10**, 93–8.

Consumer Health Information Consortium. (1994). *But will It work, doctor? Report of a conference about involving users of health services in outcomes research, held at the Kings Fund Centre on November 9th 1993*. Consumer Health Information Consortium, London.

Copperman, H. (1988). Domiciliary hospice care: a survey of general practitioners. *Journal of the Royal College of General Practitioners*, **38**, 411–13.

Corner, J. (1991). In search of more complete answers to research questions. Quantitative versus qualitative research methods: is there a way forward? *Journal of Advanced Nursing*, **16**, 718–27.

Corner, J. (1993). The nursing perspective. In *Oxford textbook of palliative medicine* (ed. D. Doyle, G. Hanks, and N. MacDonald), pp. 781–90. Oxford University Press.

Coughlan, M.C. (1993). Knowledge of diagnosis, treatment and its side-effects in patients receiving chemotherapy for cancer. *European Journal of Cancer Care*, **2**, 66–71.

Coulter, A. (1991). Evaluating the outcomes of health care. In *The sociology of the health service* (ed. J. Gabe, M. Calnan, and M. Bury), pp. 115–39. Routledge, London.

Coulter, F., *et al.* (1993). The role of lipids in the increased mortality following bereavement, (letter). *Clinica Chimica Acta*, **214**, 119–22.

Courtens, A.M., Stevens, F.C.J., Crebolder, H.F.J.M., and Philipsen, H. (1996). Longitudinal study on quality of life and social support in cancer patients. *Cancer Nursing*, **19**, 162–9.

Cronbach, L.J. (1982). *Designing evaluations of educational and social programs*. Jossey-Bass, San Francisco.

Dand, P., Field, D., Ahmedzai, S., and Biswas, B. (1991). *Client satisfaction with care at the Leicestershire Hospice*. Occasional paper no. 2. Trent Palliative Care Centre, Sheffield.

Dawson, N.J. (1991). Need satisfaction in terminal care settings. *Social Science and Medicine*, **32**, 65 and 83–6.

den Daas, N. (1995). Estimating length of survival in end-stage cancer: A review of the literature. *Journal of Pain and Symptom Management*, **10**, 548–55.

Denzin, N.K. (1988). *The research act: a theoretical introduction to sociological methods*. Prentice Hall, Englewood Cliffs, N.J.

Denzin, N.K. and Lincoln, Y.S. (1994). Introduction: entering the field of qualitative research. In *Handbook of qualitative research* (ed. N.K. Denzin and Y.S. Lincoln), pp. 1–17. Sage, Thousand Oaks.

Department of Health (1993). *Research for health*. Department of Health, London.

Donaldson, R.J. and Donaldson, L.J. (1993). *Essential public health medicine*. Kluwer, Lancaster.

Dowie, J. (1996). 'Evidence-based', 'cost-effective' and 'preference-driven' medicine: decision analysis based medical decision making is the pre-requisite. *Journal of Health Services Research and Policy*, **1**, 104–13.

Downing, G.M., Braithwaite, D.L., and Wilde, J.M. (1993). Victoria BGY Palliative Care Model—a new model for the 1990s. *Journal of Palliative Care*, **9**, 26–32.

Doyle, D. (1991). A home care service for terminally ill patients in Edinburgh. *Health Bulletin*, **49**, 14–23.

Doyle, D., Hanks, G., and MacDonald, N. (1993). Introduction. In *Oxford textbook of palliative medicine* (ed. D. Doyle, G. Hanks, and N. MacDonald), pp. 3–10. Oxford University Press.

Dudley, J.R., Smith, C., and Millison, M.B. (1995). Unfinished business: assessing the spiritual needs of hospice clients. *American Journal of Hospice and Palliative Care*, **March/April**, 30–7.

Dunphy, K.P. (1990). A comparison of hospice and home care patients; patterns of referral, patient characteristics and predictors of place of death. *Palliative Medicine*, **4**, 105–11.

Dunt, D.R., Cantwell, A.M., and Temple-Smith, M.J. (1989). The cost-effectiveness of the Citymission Hospice Programme, Melbourne. *Palliative Medicine*, 3, 125–34.

Dworkind, M., Shvartzman, P., Adler, P.S., and Franco, E.D. (1994). Urban family physicians and the care of cancer patients. *Canadian Family Physician*, 40, 47–50.

Ellershaw, J.E., Peat, S.J., and Boys, L.C. (1995). Assessing the effectiveness of a hospital palliative care team. *Palliative Medicine*, 9, 145–52.

Engel, C. (1994). A functional anatomy of teamwork. In *Going interprofessional: working together for health and welfare* (ed. A. Leathard), pp. 64–89. Routledge, London.

Eve, A. and Smith, A.M. (1994). Palliative care services in Britain and Ireland—update 1991. *Palliative Medicine*, 8, 19–27.

Eve, A., Smith, A.M., and Tebbit, P. (1997). Hospice and palliative care in the UK 1994–5, including summary of trends 1990–5. *Palliative Medicine*, 11, 31–43.

Everitt, A. and Hardiker, P. (1996). *Evaluating for good practice.* Macmillan, Basingstoke.

Expert Advisory Group on Cancer. (1995). *A policy framework for commissioning cancer services.* Department of Health, London.

Faithfull, S. (1996). How many subjects are needed in a research sample in palliative care? *Palliative Medicine*, 10, 259–61.

Faulkner, A. and O'Neill, W. (1994). Bedside manner revisited: teaching effective interaction. *European Journal of Palliative Care*, 1, 92–5.

Faulkner, A. (1992). The evaluation of training programmes for communicating skills in palliative care. *Journal of Cancer Care*, 175–8.

Ferman, L.A. (1969). Some perspectives on evaluating social welfare programs. *Annals of the American Academy of Political and Social Science*, 385, 143–56.

Ferrell, B.R., Johston Taylor, E., Sattler, G.R., Fowler, M., and Cheyney, B.L. (1993). Searching for the meaning of pain: cancer patients', caregivers', and nurses' perspectives. *Cancer Practice*, 1, 185–94.

Field, D. (1994). Client satisfaction with terminal care. *Progress in Palliative Care*, 2, 228–32.

Field, D., Dand, P., Ahmedzai, S., and Biswas, B. (1992). Care and information received by lay carers of terminally ill patients at the Leicestershire Hospice. *Palliative Medicine*, 6, 51–9.

Field, D., Douglas, C., Jagger, C., and Dand, P. (1995). Terminal illness: views of patients and their lay carers. *Palliative Medicine*, 9, 45–54.

Finch, J. and Mason, J. (1993). *Negotiating family responsibilities.* Routledge, London.

Finlay, I.G. (1993). Audit experience: views of a hospice director. In *Clinical audit in palliative care* (ed. I. Higginson), pp. 144–55. Radcliffe Medical Press, Oxford.

Finlay, I.G. and Dunlop, R. (1994). Quality of life assessment in palliative care. *Annals of Oncology*, 5, 13–18.

Finlay, I.G. and Jones, R.V.H. (1995). Definitions in palliative care (letter). *British Medical Journal*, 311, 754.

Fisher, M. (1996). How do members of an interprofessional clinical team adjust to hospice care? *Palliative Medicine*, 10, 319–28.

Fitzpatrick, R. and Boulton, M. (1994). Qualitative methods for assessing health care. *Quality in Health Care*, 3, 107–13.

Fleissig, A. and Grant, K.A.M. (1984). Transferable deaths: their epidemiological importance. *British Medical Journal*, 288, 1123.

Folkman, S. and Lazarus, R.S. (1988). *Manual of the Ways of Coping Questionnaire.* Consulting Psychologists Press, Palo Alto.

Foulstone, S., Harvey, B., Wright, J., Jay, M., Owen, F., and Cole R. (1993). Bereavement support: evaluation of a palliative care memorial service. *Palliative Medicine*, 7, 307–11.

Frankel, S.J. and Kammerling, M. (1990). Assessing the need for hospice beds. *Health Trends*, 22, 83–6.

Frankel, S.J. (1991). Health needs, health-care requirements, and the myth of infinite demand. *Lancet*, 337, 1588–90.

Gaston-Johansson, F. (1996). Measurement of pain: the psychometric properties of the Pain-O-Meter, a simple, inexpensive pain assessment tool that could change health care practices. *Journal of Pain and Symptom Management*, 12, 172–81.

Gill, L., Goldacre, M., Simmons, H., Bettley, G., and Griffith, M. (1993). Computerised linking of medical records: methodological guidelines. *Journal of Epidemiology and Community Health*, 47, 316–19.

Girling, D., Hopwood, P., and Ahmedzai, S. (1994). Assessing quality of life in palliative oncology. *Progress in Palliative Care*, 2, 80–6.

Given, C.W., Stommel, M., Given, B., Osuch, J., Kurtz, M.E., and Kurtz, J.C. (1993). The influence of cancer patients' symptoms and functional states on patients' depression and family caregivers' reaction and depression. *Health Psychology*, 12, 277–85.

Glaser, B.G. and Strauss, A.L. (1967). *The discovery of grounded theory: strategies for qualitative research.* Aldine, New York.

Glendinning, C. (1992). *The costs of informal care: looking inside the household.* HMSO, London.

Goddard, M. (1989). The role of economics in the evaluation of hospice care. *Health Policy*, 13, 19–34.

Goddard, M. (1993). The importance of assessing the effectiveness of care: the case of hospices. *Journal of Social Policy*, 22, 1–17.

Goldberg, D.P. and Williams, P. (1988). *Users guide to the General Health Questionnaire.* NFER–Nelson, Windsor.

Gordon, A.K. (1996). Hospice and minorities: A national study of organizational access and practice. *Hospice Journal*, **11**, 49–70.

Graham, H. and Livesley, B. (1983). Dying as a diagnosis: Difficulties of communication and management in elderly patients. *Lancet*, **ii**, 670–2.

Graham, J., Ramirez, A.J., Cull, A., Finlay, I., Hoy, A.,and Richards, M.A. (1996). Job stress and satisfaction among palliative care physicians. *Palliative Medicine*, **10**, 185–94.

Grassi, L., *et al.* (1996). Depressive symptoms and quality of life in home-care-assisted cancer patients. *Journal of Pain and Symptom Management*, **12**, 300–7.

Gray, D., MacAdam, D., and Boldy, D. (1987). A comparative cost analysis of terminal cancer care in home hospice patients and controls. *Journal of Chronic Diseases*, **40**, 801–10.

Greer, D.S., Mor, V., Morris, J.N., Sherwood, S., Kidder, D., and Birnbaum, H. (1986). An alternative in terminal care: results of the National Hospice Study. *Journal of Chronic Diseases*, **39**, 9–26.

Griffith, D. (1993). Respite care should be made less difficult. *British Medical Journal*, **306**, 160.

Griffith, S., Dewberry, H.M., Titcombe, J.M., McNamara, P.J.G., Harcourt, J.M.V., and Twycross, R.G. (1990). Evaluation of the palatability of Oramorph—a proprietary preparation of oral morphine sulphate. *Palliative Medicine*, **4**, 205–9.

Gullickson, C. (1993). My death nearing its future: a Heideggerian hermeneutical analysis of the lived experience of persons with chronic illness. *Journal of Advanced Nursing*, **18**, 1386–92.

Guyatt, G.H., Keller, J.L., Jaeschke, R., Rosenbloom, D., Adachi, J.D., and Newhouse, M.T. (1990). The n-of-1 randomized controlled trial: clinical usefulness. *Annals of Internal Medicine*, **112**, 293–9.

Haes, J.C.M. de, Van Knippenberg, F.C.E., and Neijt, J.P. (1990). Measuring psychological and physical distress in cancer patients: structure and application of the Rotterdam Symptom Checklist. *British Journal of Cancer*, **62**, 1034–8.

Haines, A. and Booroff, A. (1986). Terminal care at home: perspective from general practice. *British Medical Journal*, **292**, 1051–3.

Harris, R.D., Bond, M.J., and Turnbull, R. (1990). Nursing stress and stress reduction in palliative care. *Palliative Medicine*, **4**, 191–6.

Hayes, A. (1993). Audit experience: assessing staff views. In *Clinical audit in palliative care* (ed. I. Higginson), pp. 138–43. Radcliffe Medical Press, Oxford.

Herd, E.B. (1990). Terminal care in a semi-rural area. *British Journal of General Practice*, **40**, 248–51.

Herth, K. (1993). Hope in the family caregiver of terminally ill people. *Journal of Advanced Nursing*, **18**, 538–48.

Hickey, A.M., Bury, G., O'Boyle, C.A., Bradley, F., O'Kelly, F.D., and Shannon, W. (1996). A new short form individual quality of life measure (SEIQoL-DW): application in a cohort of individuals with HIV/AIDS. *British Medical Journal*, **313**, 29–33.

Higginson, I. and McCarthy, M. (1989). Evaluation of palliative care: steps to quality assurance? *Palliative Medicine*, **3**, 267–74.

Higginson,I., Wade, A., and McCarthy, M. (1990). Palliative care: views of patients and their families. *British Medical Journal*, **301**, 277–81.

Higginson, I. (1992). *Quality, standards, organizational and clinical audit for hospice and palliative care services*. NCHSPCS, London.

Higginson, I. (1993). Audit methods: a community schedule. In *Clinical audit in palliative care* (ed. I. Higginson), pp. 34–47. Radcliffe Medical Press, Oxford.

Higginson, I. and McCarthy, M. (1993). Validity of the support team assessment schedule: do staffs' ratings reflect those made by patients or their families? *Palliative Medicine*, **7**, 219–28.

Higginson, I., Priest, P., and McCarthy, M. (1994). Are bereaved family members a valid proxy for a patient's assessment of dying? *Social Science and Medicine*, **38**, 553–7.

Higginson, I. (1995). What do palliative care staff think about audit? *Journal of Palliative Care*, **11**, 17–19.

Higginson, I. (1997). Palliative and terminal care. In *Health care needs assessment: the epidemiologically based needs assessment reviews* (ed. A. Stevens and J. Raftery), pp. 1–79. Radcliffe Medical Press, Oxford.

Hill, D. and Penso, D. (1995). Opening doors: improving access to hospice and specialist palliative care services by members of the black and ethnic minority communities. NCHSPCS, London.

Hill, F. and Oliver, C. (1984). Hospice—the cost of in-patient care. *Health Trends*, **16**, 9–11.

Hill, F., Oliver, C. (1989). Hospice—an update on the cost of patient care. *Palliative Medicine*, **3**, 119–24.

Hinton, J. (1994). Can home care maintain an acceptable quality of life for patients with terminal cancer and their relatives? *Palliative Medicine*, **8**, 183–96.

Hinton, J. (1996). How reliable are relatives' retrospective reports of terminal illness? Patients' and relatives' accounts compared. *Social Science and Medicine*, **43**, 1229–36.

Hockey, J.L. (1990). *Experiences of death: an anthropological account*. Edinburgh University Press.

Hockey, L. (1991). St Columba's Hospice Home Care Service: an evaluation study. *Palliative Medicine*, **5**, 315–22.

Hogan, N., Morse, J.M., and Tasón, M.C. (1996). Toward an experiential theory of bereavement. *Omega*, **33**, 43–65.

Holland, W.W. (1983). *Evaluation of health care*. Oxford University Press.

Holman, H.R. (1993). Qualitative inquiry in medical research. *Journal of Clinical Epidemiology*, **46**, 29–36.

Hospice Information Service. (1997). 1997 directory of hospice and palliative care services. Hospice Information Service, at St Christopher's Hospice.

Huberman, A.M. and Miles, M.B. (1994). Data management and analysis methods, In *Handbook of qualitative research* (ed. N.K. Denzin and Y.S. Lincoln), pp. 428–444. Sage, Thousand Oaks.

Hunt, M. (1991). The identification and provision of care for the terminally ill at home by 'family' members. *Sociology of Health and Illness*, **13**, 375–95.

Hunt, S., McKenna, S.P., McEwen, J., Williams J., and Papp, E. (1981). The Nottingham Health Profile: subjective health status and medical consultations. *Social Science and Medicine*, **15A**, 221–9.

Ingleton, C. and Faulkner, A. (1993). Audit issues in palliative care: the perspective of senior nurses. *Journal of Cancer Care*, **2**, 201–6.

Jacobs, S., Kasl, S., Ostfeld, A., Berkman, L., Kosten, T., and Charpentier, P. (1986). The measurement of grief: bereaved versus non-bereaved. *Hospice Journal*, **2**, 21–36.

James, M.L., Gebski, V.J., and Gunz, F.W. (1985). The need for palliative care services in a general hospital. *Medical Journal of Australia*, **142**, 448–9.

James, N. (1992). Care = organisation + physical labour + emotional labour. *Sociology of Health and Illness*, **14**, 488–509.

Jamison, R.N. (1996). Comprehensive pretreatment and outcome assessment for chronic opioid therapy in nonmalignant pain. *Journal of Pain and Symptom Management*, **11**, 231–41.

Jarvis, H., Burge, F.I., Scott, C.A. (1996). Evaluating a palliative care program: methodology and limitations. *Journal of Palliative Care*, **12**, 23–33.

Jeffreys, D. (1994) Education in palliative care: a qualitative evaluation of the present state and the needs of general practitioners and community nurses. *European Journal of Cancer Care*, **3**, 67–74.

Jenkins, H. (1989). The family and loss: a systems framework. *Palliative Medicine*, **3**, 97–104.

Johnson, H. and Oliver, D. (1991). The development of palliative care services and the place of death of cancer patients. *Palliative Medicine*, **5**, 40–5.

Johnson, J.R. and Miller, A.J. (1994). The efficacy of choline magnesium trisalicylate (CMT) in the management of metastatic bone pain: a pilot study. *Palliative Medicine*, 8, 129–35.

Johnson, I.S., Rogers, C., Biswas, B., and Ahmedzai, S. (1990). What do hospices do? A survey of hospices in the United Kingdom. *British Medical Journal*, 300, 791–3.

Johnston, G. and Abraham, C. (1995). The WHO objectives for palliative care: to what extent are we achieving them? *Palliative Medicine*, 9, 123–37.

Jones, D.A. and Peters, T.J. (1992). Caring for elderly dependants: Effects on the carers' quality of life. *Age and Ageing*, 21, 421–8.

Jones, R.V.H. (1995). Improving terminal care at home: can district nurses act as catalysts? *European Journal of Cancer Care*, 4, 80–5.

Jones, R.V.H., Hansford, J., and Fiske, J. (1993). Death from cancer at home: the carers' perspective. *British Medical Journal*, 306, 249–51.

Kaasa, T., Loomis, J., Gillis, K., Bruera, and E., Hanson, J. (1997). The Edmonton Functional Assessment Tool: preliminary development and evaluation for use in palliative care. *Journal of Pain and Symptom Management*, 13, 10–19.

Kagawa-Singer, M. (1993). Redefining health: living with cancer. *Social Science and Medicine*, 37, 295–304.

Kane, R.L., Wales, J., Berstein. L. Leibowitz A., and Kaplan, S. (1984). A randomized controlled trial of hospice care. *Lancet*, i, 890–5.

Kane, R.L. (1986). Lessons from hospice evaluations. *Hospice Journal*, 2, 3–8.

Karnofsky, D.A. and Burchenal, J.H. (1949). The clinical evaluation of chemotherapeutic agents in cancer, In *Evaluation of chemotherapeutic agents*. (ed. C.M. Macleod), pp. 191–205. Columbia University Press, New York.

Kay, M., Zapien, J.G., Wilson, C.A., and Yoder, M. (1993). Evaluating treatment efficacy by triangulation. *Social Science and Medicine*, 36, 1545–54.

Keane, W.G., Gould, J.H., and Millard, P.H. (1983). Death in practice. *Journal of the Royal College of General Practitioners*, 33, 347–51.

Kidder, D. (1988). The impact of hospices on the health-care costs of terminal cancer patients, In *The hospice experiment* (ed. V. Mor, D.S. Greer, and R. Kastenbaum), pp. 48–68. John Hopkins University Press, Baltimore.

Kind, P. (1988). *Hospital deaths—the missing link: measuring outcome in hospital activity data*. Discussion paper 4, Centre for Health Economics, University of York.

King, C.R., *et al*. (1997). Quality of life and the cancer experience: the state-of-the-knowledge. *Oncology Nursing Forum*, 24, 27–41.

King, M., Lapsley, I., Llewellyn, S., Tierney, A., Anderson, J., and Sladden, S. (1993). Purchasing palliative care: Availability and cost implications. *Health Bulletin*, **51**, 370–384.

Kiresuk, T.J. and Sherman, R.E. (1968). Goal attainment scaling: a general method for evaluating community mental health programs. *Community Mental Health Journal*, **4**, 443–53.

Kirkham, S. and Davis, M. (1992). Bed occupancy, patient throughput and size of independent hospice units in the UK. *Palliative Medicine*, **6**, 47–53.

Kirschling, J.M. and Pittman, J.F. (1989). Measurement of spiritual well-being: a hospice caregiver sample. *Hospice Journal*, **5**, 1–11.

Komesaroff, P.A., Moss, C.K., and Fox, R.M. (1989). Patients' socio-economic background: influence on selection of inpatient or domiciliary hospice terminal-care programmes. *Medical Journal of Australia*, **151**, 196–201.

Krefting, L. and Krefting, D. (1991). Leisure activities after a stroke: An ethnographic approach. *American Journal of Occupational Therapy*, **45**, 429–36.

Kristjanson, L.J. (1989). Quality of terminal care: salient indicators identified by families. *Journal of Palliative Care*, **5**, 21–8.

Kristjanson, L.J. (1993), Validity and reliability testing of the FAMCARE Scale: measuring family satisfaction with advanced cancer care. *Social Science and Medicine*, **36**, 693–701.

Kristjanson, L.J. (1994). Research in palliative care populations: Ethical issues. *Journal of Palliative Care*, **10**, 10–15.

Kristjanson, L., Sloan, J.A., Dudgeon, D., and Adaskin, E. (1996). Family members' perceptions of palliative cancer care: predictors of family functioning and family members' health. *Journal of Palliative Care*, **12**, 10–20.

Lewis, J. (1994). Voluntary organizations in "New Partnership" with local authorities: the anatomy of a contract. *Social Policy and Administration*, **28**, 206–20.

Lichter, I., Mooney, J., and Boyd, M. (1993). Biography as therapy. *Palliative Medicine*, **7**, 133–7.

Lieberman, M.A. and Yalom, I. (1992). Brief group psychotherapy for the spousally bereaved: a controlled study. *International Journal of Group Psychotherapy*, **42**, 117–32.

Ling, J. and Penn, K. (1995). The challenges of conducting clinical trials in palliative care. *International Journal of Palliative Nursing*, **1**, 31–4.

Littlewood, J.L. (1992). *Aspects of grief*. Routledge, London.

Lunt, B. and Hillier, R. (1981). Terminal care: present services and future priorities. *British Medical Journal*, **283**, 595–8.

Lunt, B. and Neale, C. (1987). A comparison of hospice and hospital: care goals set by staff. *Palliative Medicine*, 1, 136–48.

Lydick, E. and Epstein, R.S. (1993). Interpretation of quality of life changes. *Quality of Life Research*, 2, 221–6.

Lynch, J., Zech, D., and Grond, S. (1992). The role of intrathecal neurolysis in the treatment of cancer-related perianal and perineal pain. *Palliative Medicine*, 6, 140–5.

MacAdam, D.B. and Smith, M. (1987). An initial assessment of suffering in terminal illness. *Palliative Medicine*, 1, 37–47.

Macdonald, E.T. and Macdonald, J.B. (1992). How do local doctors react to a hospice? *Health Bulletin*, 50, 351–5.

MacDonald, N. (1993). Ontario palliative care statement: a template for the rest of Canada. *Canadian Medical Association Journal*, 148, 891–3.

Macleod, R.D., Nash, A., and Charny, M. (1994). Evaluating palliative care education. *European Journal of Cancer Care*, 3, 163–8.

Mah, M.A. and Johnston, C. (1993). Concerns of families in which one member has head and neck cancer. *Cancer Nursing*, 16, 382–7.

Maltoni, M., Pirovano, M., Nanni, O., Labianca, R., and Amadori, D. (1994). Prognostic factors in terminal cancer patients. *European Journal of Palliative Care*, 1, 122–5.

Marquis, R. (1996). A qualitative evaluation of a bereavement service: An analysis of the experiences of consumers and providers of services in Australia. *American Journal of Hospice and Palliative Care*, **July/August**, 38–43.

Maturana, A.L. de, Morago, V., San Emeterio, E., Gorostiza, J., and Arrate, A.O. (1993). Attitudes of general practitioners in Bizkaia, Spain, towards the terminally ill patient. *Palliative Medicine*, 7, 39–45.

Maudsley, G. and Williams, E.M.I. (1996). 'Inaccuracy' in death certification—where are we now? *Journal of Public Health Medicine*, 18, 59–66.

McCorkle, R. and Young, K. (1978). Development of a symptom distress scale. *Cancer Nursing*, 1, 373–8.

McGourty, H. (1993). *How to evaluate complementary therapies: a literature review*. Liverpool Public Health Observatory.

McMillan, S.C. (1996). The quality of life of patients with cancer receiving hospice care. *Oncology Nursing Forum*, 23, 1221–8.

McNair, D.M., Lorr, M., and Droppleman, L.F. (1992). *EdITS manual for the Profile of Mood States (POMS)*. EdITS/Educational and Industrial Testing Service, San Diego.

McQuay, H. and Moore, A. (1994). Need for rigorous assessment of palliative care. *British Medical Journal*, 309, 1315–16.

McQuillan, R., Finlay, I., Roberts, D., Branch, C., Forbes, F., and Spencer, M.G. (1996). The provision of a palliative care service in a teaching hospital and subsequent evaluation of that service. *Palliative Medicine*, **10**, 213–19.

McWhinney, I.R. and Stewart, M.A. (1994a). Home care of dying patients: Family physicians' experience with a palliative care support team. *Canadian Family Physician*, **40**, 240–6.

McWhinney, I.R., Bass, M.J., and Donner, A. (1994). Evaluation of a palliative care service: problems and pitfalls. *British Medical Journal*, **309**, 1340–2.

Melzack, R. (1987). The short-form McGill Pain Questionnaire. *Pain*, **30**, 191–17.

Millison, M.B. (1995). A review of the research on spiritual care and hospice. *The Hospice Journal*, **10**, 3–18.

Mills, M., Davies, H.T.O., and Macrae, W.A. (1994). Care of dying patients in hospital. *British Medical Journal*, **309**, 583–6.

Millward, L. (1995). Focus groups. In Research methods in psychology (ed. G.M. Breakwell, S. Hammond, and C. Fife-Schaw), pp. 274–92. Sage, London.

Montazeri, A., Gillis, C.R., and McEwen, J. (1996*a*). Measuring quality of life in oncology: is it worthwhile? I. Meaning, purposes and controversies. *European Journal of Cancer Care*, **5**, 159–67.

Montazeri, A., Gillis, C.R., and McEwen, J. (1996*b*). Measuring quality of life in oncology: is it worthwhile? II. Experiences from the treatment of cancer. *European Journal of Cancer Care*, **5**, 168–75.

Moore, M.K. (1993). Dying at home: a way of maintaining control for the person with ALS/MND. *Palliative Medicine*, **7** (suppl 2), 65–8.

Mor, V. (1988). The research design of the National Hospice Study. In *The hospice experiment* (ed. V. Mor, D.S. Greer, and R. Kastenbaum), pp. 28–47. John Hopkins University Press, Baltimore.

Mount, B.M. (1976). The problem of caring for the dying in a general hospital; the palliative care unit as a possible solution. *Canadian Medical Association Journal*, **115**, 119–21.

Mount, B.M. and Scott, J.F. (1983). Whither hospice evaluation? *Journal of Chronic Diseases*, **36**, 731–6.

Mount, B.M., Cohen, R., MacDonald, N., Bruera, E., and Dudgeon, D. (1995). Ethical issues in palliative care research revisited. (Letter) *Palliative Medicine*, **9**, 165–70.

Murray, D.B. (1993). Education and training of clergy in palliative care. In *Oxford textbook of palliative medicine* (ed. D. Doyle, G. Hanks, and N. MacDonald), pp. 795–9. Oxford University Press.

Nash, A. and Hoy, A. (1993). Terminal care in the community— an evaluation of residential workshops for general practitioner/district nurse teams. *Palliative Medicine*, **7**, 5–17.

National Association of Health Authorities and Trusts. (1991). *Care of people with terminal illness*. Birmingham.

NCHSPCS (1994). Minister replies to council concern over funding. *Information Exchange*, 9, 20.

NCHSPCS (1995a). *Specialist palliative care: a statement of definitions*. Occasional paper 8. London.

NCHSPCS (1995b). *Guidelines on research in palliative care*. London.

NCHSPCS (1995c). Progress on national information project. *Information Exchange*, 13, 4.

Neale, B. (1991). *Informal palliative care: a review of research in needs, standards and service evaluation*. Occasional paper no. 3. Trent Palliative Care Centre, Sheffield.

Neale, B., Clark, D., and Heather, P. (1993). *Purchasing palliative care: a review of the policy and research literature*. Occasional paper no. 11. Trent Palliative Care Centre, Sheffield.

Norman, I., Redfern, S., Tomalin, D., and Oliver, S. (1992). Applying triangulation to the assessment of quality of nursing. *Nursing Times*, 88, 43–6.

Normand, C. (1996). Economics and evaluation of palliative care. *Palliative Medicine*, 10, 3–4.

Nuland, S.B. (1997). *How we die*, p. 268. Vintage, London.

Ong, B.N. (1993). *The practice of health services research*, p. 105. Chapman and Hall, London.

OPCS (1992). Mortality statistics: general (England and Wales). Series DH1 no. 27. HMSO.

Orchard, C. (1994). Comparing outcomes. *British Medical Journal*, 308, 1493–6.

Padilla, G.V., Mishel, M.H., and Grant, M.M. (1992) Uncertainty, appraisal and quality of life. *Quality of Life Research*, 1, 155–65.

Parkes, C.M. (1978). Home or hospital? Terminal care as seen by surviving spouses. *Journal of the Royal College of General Practitioners*, 28, 19–30.

Parkes, C.M. (1981). Evaluation of a bereavement service. *Journal of Preventive Psychiatry*, 1, 179–88.

Parkes, C.M. (1986). *Bereavement: studies of grief in adult life*. Penguin, Harmondsworth.

Parkes, C.M. (1993a). Bereavement. In *Oxford textbook of palliative medicine* (ed. D. Doyle, G. Hanks, and N. MacDonald), pp. 665–78. Oxford University Press.

Parkes, C.M. (1993b). Psychiatric problems following bereavement by murder or manslaughter. *British Journal of Psychiatry*, 162, 49–54.

Partridge, M. (1989). NHS provision for terminal care: one district's deliberation. *Journal of Management in Medicine*, 3, 362–71.

Payne, S.A. and Relf, M. (1994). The assessment of need for bereavement follow-up in palliative and hospice care. *Palliative Medicine*, 8, 291–7.

Payne, S.A., Langley-Evans, A., and Hillier, R. (1996). Perceptions of a 'good' death: a comparative study of the views of hospice staff and patients. *Palliative Medicine*, 10, 307–12.

Peruselli, C., Camporesi, E., Colombo, A.M., Cucci, M., Mazzoni, G., and Paci, E. (1993). Quality of life assessment in a home care program for advanced cancer patients: a study using the symptom distress scale. *Journal of Pain and Symptom Management*, 8, 306–11.

Peräkylä, A. (1989). Appealing to the 'experience' of the patient in the care of the dying. *Sociology of Health and Illness*, 11, 117–34.

Pocock, S.J. (1983). *Clinical trials: a practical approach.* John Wiley & Sons, Chichester.

Pope, C. and Mays, N. (1995). Reaching the parts other methods cannot reach: an introduction to qualitative methods in health and health services research. *British Medical Journal*, 311, 42–5.

Pottinger, A.M. (1991). Grieving relatives' perception of their needs and adjustment in a continuing care unit. *Palliative Medicine*, 5, 117–21.

Prior, L. (1989). *The social organization of death.* Macmillan, Basingstoke.

Prouse, M. (1994). Organisational audit for palliative care services. *European Journal of Palliative Care*, 1, 184–6.

Pugsley, R. and Pardoe, J. (1986). The specialist contribution to the care of the terminally ill patients: support or substitution? *Journal of the Royal College of General Practitioners*, 36, 347–8.

Raeve, L. de, (1994). Ethical issues in palliative care research. *Palliative Medicine*, 8, 298–305.

Raftery, J., et al. (1996). A randomized controlled trial of the cost-effectiveness of a district co-ordinating service for terminally ill cancer patients. *Palliative Medicine*, 10, 151–61.

Raphael, B. (1977). Preventive intervention with the recently bereaved. *Archives of General Psychiatry*, 34, 1450.

Rathbone, G.V., Horsley, S., and Goacher, J. (1994). A self-evaluated assessment suitable for seriously ill hospice patients. *Palliative Medicine*, 8, 29–34.

Raudonis, B.M. (1992). Ethical considerations in qualitative research with hospice patients. *Qualitative Health Research*, 2, 238–49.

Raudonis, B.M. (1993). The meaning and impact of empathic relationships in hospice nursing. *Cancer Nursing*, 16, 304–9.

Redman, S., White, K., Ryan E., and Hennrikus, D. (1995). Professionals needs of palliative care nurses in New South Wales. *Palliative Medicine*, 9, 36–44.

Rees, D. and Lutkins, S. (1967). Mortality of bereavement. *British Medical Journal*, iv, 13–16.

Reese, D.J. and Brown, D.R. (1997). Psychosocial and spiritual care in hospice: differences between nursing, social work and clergy. *The Hospice Journal*, **12**, 29–41.

Richards, M.A. and Ramirez, A.J. (1997). Quality of life: the main outcome measure of palliative care. *Palliative Medicine*, **11**, 89–92.

Richards, W.R., Burgess, D.E., Petersen, F.R., and McCarthy, D.L. (1993). Genograms: a psychosocial assessment tool. *Hospice Journal*, **9**, 1–12.

Rinck, G.C., van den Bos, G.A.M., Kleijnen, J, de Haes, H.J.C, Schadé, E., and Veenhof, C.H.N. (1997). Methodologic issues in effectiveness research on palliative cancer care: a systematic review. *Journal of Clinical Oncology*, **15**, 1697–707.

Ritchie, J. and Spencer, L. (1994) Qualitative data analysis for applied policy research. In *Analyzing qualitative data* (ed. A. Bryman and R.G. Burgess), pp. 173–94. Routledge, London.

Robbins, M., Jackson, P., and Prentice, A. (1994*a*). *Palliative cancer care provision in the South West*. Health Care Evaluation Unit, University of Bristol.

Robbins, M., *et al.* (1994*b*). *Palliative care provision in Bristol and District*. Unpublished, figures available from M. Robbins, Department of Palliative Medicine, University of Bristol.

Robbins, M. and Frankel, S. (1995). Palliative care services: what needs assessment? *Palliative Medicine*, **9**, 287–93.

Robbins, M., Jackson, P., and Prentice, A. (1996*a*). Statutory and voluntary sector palliative care in the community setting: National Health Service professionals' perceptions of the interface. *European Journal of Cancer Care*, **5**, 96–102.

Robbins, M., Jackson, P., Brooks, J., and Frankel, S. (1996*b*) Framing the sample in palliative care research: reflections from one district. Research abstract. *Palliative Medicine*, **10**, 55.

Robson, C. (1993). *Real world research: a resource for social scientists and practitioner-researchers*. Blackwell, Oxford.

Room, G. (1986). *Cross-national innovation in social policy*. Macmillan, London.

Rose, G. (1995). *Love's work*, p. 110. Chatto and Windus, London.

Rosenthal, M.A., Gebski, V.J., Kefford, R.F., and Stuart-Harris, R.C. (1993). Prediction of life-expectancy in hospice patients: identification of novel prognostic factors. *Palliative Medicine*, **7**, 199–204.

Ross, M.M., Rosenthal, C.J., and Dawson, P.G. (1993). Spousal caregiving following institutionalization: the experience of elderly wives. *Journal of Advanced Nursing*, **18**, 1531–39.

Rossi, P.H. and Freeman, H.E. (1993). *Evaluation: a systematic approach*. Sage, Newbury Park.

Royal College of Physicians. (1991). *Palliative care: guidelines for good practice and audit measures*. Report of the working group of the research unit of the Royal College of Physicians, London.

Rustøen, T. (1995). Hope and quality of life, two central issues for cancer patients: a theoretical analysis. *Cancer Nursing*, **18**, 355–61.

Ruta, D.A., Garratt, A.M., Leng, M., Russell, I., and MacDonald, L.M. (1994) A new approach to the measurement of quality of life. The Patient Generated Index. *Medical Care*, **32**, 1109–26.

Sackett, D.L. (2 June 1995). *n-of-1 trials*. Via the mailbase electronic discussion list: evidence based health (evidence-based-health@mailbase.ac.uk)

Sackett, D.L. and Rosenberg, M.C. (1995). On the need for evidence-based medicine. *Journal of Public Health Medicine*, **17**, 330–4.

Sadler, I.N., West, S.G., and Baca, L. (1992). Linking empirically based theory and evaluation: The Family Bereavement Program. *American Journal of Community Psychology*, **20**, 491–521.

Saunders, C. (1993). Foreword. In *Oxford textbook of palliative medicine* (ed. D. Doyle, G. Hanks, and N. MacDonald), pp. v–ix. Oxford University Press.

Schaerer, R. (1993). Suffering of the doctor linked with the death of patients. *Palliative Medicine*, **7** (suppl 1), 27–37.

Schipper, H., Clinch, J., McMurray, A., and Levitt, M. (1984). Measuring the quality of life of cancer patients: the Functional Living Index— Cancer. Development and validation. *Journal of Clinical Oncology*, **2**, 472–83.

Scott, J.F. and MacDonald, N. (1993). Education in palliative medicine. In *Oxford textbook of palliative medicine* (ed. D. Doyle, G. Hanks, and N. MacDonald), pp. 761–80. Oxford University Press.

Seale, C. (1989). What happens in hospices: a review of the research evidence. *Social Science and Medicine*, **28**, 551–9.

Seale, C. (1991). Death from cancer and death from other causes: the relevance of the hospice approach. *Palliative Medicine*, **5**, 12–19.

Seale, C. (1995). Dying alone. *Sociology of Health and Illness*, **17**, 376–92.

Seale, C. and Kelly, M. (1997). A comparison of hospice and hospital care for the spouses of people who die. *Palliative Medicine*, **11**, 101–6.

Seamark, D.A., Thorne, C.P., Jones, R.V.H., Pereira Gray, D.J., and Searle, J.F. (1993). Knowledge and perceptions of a domiciliary hospice service among general practitioners and community nurses. *British Journal of General Practice*, **43**, 57–9.

Seamark, D.A., Thorne, C.P., Lawrence, C., and Pereira Gray, D.J. (1995). Appropriate place of death for cancer patients: views of general practitioners and hospital doctors. *British Journal of General Practice*, **45**, 359–63.

Selby, P. (1993). The value of quality of life scores in clinical cancer research. *European Journal of Cancer*, **29A**, 1656–7.

Severs, M.P. and Wilkins, P.S.W. (1991). A hospital palliative care ward for elderly people. *Age and Ageing*, **20**, 361–4.

Shanks, J. (1993). Asking patients about their treatment, (letter). *British Medical Journal*, **306**, 65.

Shaw, C. (1993). Introduction to audit in palliative care. In *Clinical audit in palliative care* (ed. I. Higginson), pp. 1–7. Radcliffe Medical Press, Oxford.

Sheldon, F. (1993). Education and training for social workers in palliative care. In *Oxford textbook of palliative medicine* (ed. D. Doyle, G. Hanks, and N. MacDonald), pp. 791–5. Oxford University Press.

Sheldon, F., Smith, P. (1996). The life so short, the craft so hard to learn: a model for post-basic education in palliative care. *Palliative Medicine*, **10**, 99–104.

Sherwood, S., Kastenbaum, R., Morris, J.N., and Wright, S.M. (1988). The months of bereavement. In *The hospice experiment* (ed. V. Mor, D.S. Greer, and R. Kastenbaum), pp. 147–86. John Hopkins University Press, Baltimore.

Sibbald, B. and Simpson, J. (1991). General practitioners' opinions of hospice care. *British Journal of General Practice*, **41**, 213–14.

Simpson, M.A. (1976). Planning for terminal care. *Lancet*, ii, 192–3.

Smith, A.M., Eve, A., and Sykes, N.P. (1992). Palliative care services in Britain and Ireland 1990—an overview. *Palliative Medicine*, **6**, 277–91.

Smith, G. and Cantley, C. (1985). *Assessing health care: a study in organizational evaluation*. Open University Press, Milton Keynes.

Smith, N. (1990). The impact of terminal illness on the family. *Palliative Medicine*, **4**, 127–35.

Smith, N. and Regnard, C. (1993). Managing family problems in advanced disease—a flow diagram. *Palliative Medicine*, **7**, 47–58.

Speer, D.C., Robinson, B.E., and Reed, M.P. (1995). The relationship between hospice length of stay and caregiver adjustment. *The Hospice Journal*, **10**, 45–58.

Spicker, P. (1995). *Social policy: themes and approaches*. Prentice Hall, London.

Spiller, J.A. and Alexander, D.A. (1993). Domiciliary care: a comparison of the views of terminally ill patients and their family caregivers. *Palliative Medicine*, **7**, 109–15.

Spitzer, W.O., *et al.* (1981). Measuring the quality of life of cancer patients. A concise QL–index for use by physicians. *Journal of Chronic Diseases*, **34**, 585–98.

Spurrell, M.T. and Creed, F.H. (1993). Lymphocyte response in depressed patients and subjects anticipating bereavement. *British Journal of Psychiatry*, **162**, 60–4.

Standing Medical Advisory Committee and Standing Nursing and Midwifery Advisory Committee (1992). *The principles and provision of palliative care*. HMSO, London.

Stecher, B.M. and Davis, W.A. (1987). *How to focus an evaluation*. Sage, California.

Steinmetz, D. and Gabel, L.L. (1992). The family physician's role in caring for the dying patient and family: a comprehensive theoretical model. *Family Practice*, 9, 433–6.

Sterkenburg, C.A. and Woodward, C.A. (1996). A reliability and validity study of the McMaster Quality of Life Scale (MQLS) for a palliative population. *Journal of Palliative Care*, 12, 18–25.

Stevens, A. and Raftery, J. (1994). *Health care needs assessment: the epidemiologically based needs assessment reviews*. Volumes 1 and 2. Radcliffe Medical Press, Oxford.

St Leger, A.S., Schnieden, H., and Walsworth-Bell, J.P. (1992). *Evaluating health services' effectiveness*. Open University Press, Milton Keynes.

Strause, L., Herbst, L., Ryndes, T., Callaghan, M., and Piro, L. (1993). A severity index designed as an indicator of acuity in palliative care. *Journal of Palliative Care*, 9, 11–15.

Streiner, D.L. and Norman, G.R. (1989). Health measurement scales: a practical guide to their development and use. Oxford University Press.

Stroebe, W. and Stroebe, M.S. (1987). *Bereavement and health: the psychological and physical consequences of partner loss*. Cambridge University Press.

Sykes, N.P., Pearson, S., and Chell, S. (1992). Quality of care of the terminally ill: the carer's perspective. *Palliative Medicine*, 6, 227–36.

Tamburini, M., Brunelli, C., Rosso, S., and Ventafridda, V. (1996). Prognostic value of quality of life scores in terminal cancer patients. *Journal of Pain and Symptom Management*, 11, 32–41.

Tierney, A.J., Sladden, S., Anderson, J., King, M., Lapsley, I., and Llewellyn, S. (1994). Measuring the costs and quality of palliative care: a discussion paper. *Palliative Medicine*, 8, 273–281.

Tigges, K.N. (1993). Quality of life: reality of rhetoric? *Loss and Grief Care*, 7, 157–67.

Thorne, C.P., Seamark, D.A., Lawrence, C., and Pereira Gray, D.J. (1994). The influence of general practitioner community hospitals on the place of death of cancer patients. *Palliative Medicine*, 8, 122–8.

Thornton, H.M. (1992). Breast cancer trials: a patient's viewpoint. *Lancet*, 339, 44–5.

Torrens, P.R. (1985). Hospice care: what have we learned? *Annual Review of Public Health*, 6, 65–83.

Townsend, J., *et al.* (1990). Terminal cancer care and patients' preference for place of death: a prospective study. *British Medical Journal*, 301, 415–17.

Traylen, H. (1994). Confronting hidden agendas: co-operative inquiry with health visitors. In *Participation in human inquiry* (ed. P. Reason), pp. 59–81. Sage, London.

Trent Hospice Audit Group. (1992). *Palliative care core standards: a multidisciplinary approach.* Derbyshire Royal Infirmary, UK.

Twycross, R.G. and Dunn, V. (1994). *Research in palliative care: the pursuit of reliable knowledge.* NCHSPCS, London.

Twycross, R., Harcourt, J., and Bergl, S. (1996). A survey of pain in patients with advanced cancer. *Journal of Pain and Symptom Management*, 12, 273–82.

Vachon, M.L.S. (1995). Staff stress in hospice / palliative care: a review. *Palliative Medicine*, 9, 91–122.

Vachon, M.L.S., Kristjanson, L., and Higginson, I. (1995). Psychosocial issues in palliative care: the patient, the family, and the process and outcome of care. *Journal of Pain and Symptom Management*, 10, 142–50.

Vainio, A. (1993). Symptom evaluation in cancer care. *Progress in Palliative Care*, 1, 51–3.

Vainio, A., *et al.* (1996). Prevalence of symptoms among patients with advanced cancer: an international collaborative study. *Journal of Pain and Symptom Management*, 12, 3–10.

Ventafridda, V., De Conno, F., Viganò, A., Ripamonti, C., Gallucci, M., and Gamba, A. (1989). Comparison of home and hospital care of advanced cancer patients. *Tumori*, 75, 619–625.

Ventafridda, V., De Conno, F., Ripamonti, C., Gamba, A., and Tamburini, M. (1990). Quality-of-life assessment during a palliative care programme. *Annals of Oncology*, 1, 415–20.

Wakefield, M. and Ashby, M. (1993). Attitudes of surviving relatives to terminal care in South Australia. *Journal of Pain and Symptom Management*, 8, 529–37.

Wakefield, M.A., Beilby, J., and Ashby, M.A. (1993). General practitioners and palliative care. *Palliative Medicine*, 7, 117–26.

Walter, T. (1994). *The revival of death*, pp. 47–65. Routledge, London.

Ware, J. and Sherbourne, C.D. (1992). The MOS 36–item short form health survey (SF-36): conceptual framework and item selection. *Medical Care*, 30, 473–81.

Weiss, C. (1979). The many meanings of research utilisation. *Public Administration Review*, 39, 426–31.

Weiss, R.S. and Rein, M. (1969). The evaluation of broad-aim programs: a cautionary case and a moral. *Annals of the American Academy of Political and Social Science*, 385, 133–42.

WHO Expert Committee. (1990). *Cancer pain relief and palliative care*, Technical report series 804. World Health Organization, Geneva.

Wilkes, E. (1965). Terminal cancer at home. *Lancet*, **i**, 799–801.

Wilkes, E. (1993). Characteristics of hospice bereavement services. *Journal of Cancer Care*, **2**, 183–9.

Williams, A. (1995). Dependency scoring in palliative care. *Nursing Standard*, **10**, 27–30.

Wilson, I.M., Bunting, J.S., Curnow, R.N., and Knock, J. (1995). The need for inpatient palliative care facilities for noncancer patients in the Thames Valley. *Palliative Medicine*, **9**, 13–18.

Yang, C-T. and Kirschling, J.M. (1992). Exploration of factors related to direct care and outcomes of caregiving: Caregivers of terminally ill older persons. *Cancer Nursing*, **15**, 173–81.

Youll, J.W. (1989). The bridge beyond: strengthening nursing practice in attitudes towards death, dying, and the terminally ill, and helping the spouses of critically ill patients. *Intensive Care Nursing*, **5**, 88–94.

Zalot, G.N. (1989). Planning a regional palliative care services network. *Journal of Palliative Care*, **5**, 42–6.

Zigmond, A.S. and Snaith, R.R. (1983). The Hospital Anxiety and Depression scale. *Acta Psychiatrica Scandinavica*, **67**, 361–70

Zubrod, C.G., *et al.* (1960). Appraisal of methods for the study of chemotherapy of cancer in man: comparative therapeutic trial of nitrogen mustard and triethylene thiophosphoramide. *Journal of Chronic Diseases*, **11**, 7–33.

Zung, W.W.K. (1965). A self-rating depression scale. *Archives of General Psychiatry*, **16**, 543–7.

Index